BRONCO PORTER

1-Minute Wall Pilates Workouts For Busy Women

On-The-Go Guided Exercises To Sculpt Abs & Glutes, Anywhere, Anytime

Contents

I

Introducing 1-Minute Wall Pilates

The Gateway Exercise Book for Busy Women On-The-Go

Hey there! Bronco here. I'm so thrilled you've picked up this exercise guide. I promise this won't take a lot of time – just get through this one chapter and we will get straight to the good stuff. I need to talk about something that's a game-changer for all you busy bees out there – Wall Pilates. You see, in our whirlwind lives, squeezing in time for a workout feels like a Herculean task. But guess what? Wall Pilates is about to make your fitness journey not just possible, but incredibly effective.

Why Wall Pilates? Let Me Tell You.

Think of Wall Pilates as your fitness hack. It's not just another exercise; it's a revolution in how we think about staying fit amid chaos. Here's the deal – it's quick, flexible, and oh-so-rewarding. Why is it the best though, you ask? Pull up a chair (or wall), and let's dive into the reasons why Wall Pilates will become your new best friend.

The Magic of Wall Pilates

Picture this: an exercise routine that molds to your impossibly packed schedule and still gives you those visible gains, fast. That's Wall Pilates for you. Here's what's in store:

- **Time-Saver:** Got a minute? That's all you need to kickstart your routine.
- **No Space, No Problem:** All you need is a wall. Seriously, that's it.
- **Core Power:** A few sessions in, and you'll feel that core tightening up – the cornerstone of a strong physique.
- **Glute Sculpting:** Get ready for lifted and toned glutes that make every pair of jeans your favorite.
- **Stand Tall:** Wave goodbye to slouching. Improved posture and flexibility are on the horizon.
- **Stress, Be Gone:** Notice your stress levels dropping and your mental clarity soaring.

So Wall Pilates is magical, are you getting the picture? But here's the thing - it comes down to you to find that out for yourself. You may have some doubts, but look past them and please just make the commitment to do this – right now. Listen, I'm not asking for the sun, the moon, and the stars. It's just 1-minute. And we both know you have *that* 1-minute - okay, let's stop pretending here, you have a lot more time than 1-minute.

If it isn't clear by now, this isn't a book about making health your singular priority, but with that said, health should be a serious priority somewhere in your long list of life goals. Because if it is a priority and you carve out the smallest amount of time in the right direction, then will witness how even the briefest sessions can lead to significant changes. The type of changes I am talking about are not just in how you look, but in how you feel and carry yourself through life's rush. Let's make every minute count!

How to Use This Guide

This book is your straightforward path to getting moving, pronto. It's all about making Pilates far more accessible and faster to get results. It doesn't matter if you're a newbie or if you've been at this fitness game for a while; there's something in here for everyone:

- **Levels for All:** Beginner, intermediate, advanced – take your pick and progress at your pace.
- **Focus on What Matters:** Targeted workouts mean you can hone in on specific muscle groups.
- **You Set the Intensity:** From a gentle stretch to a full-on workout, you're in control - you can skip around within a given workout.

The Essence of 1-Minute Wall Pilates

Here's the thing: even a single minute can set you on the path to a healthier you. Got 3-5 minutes? Perfect. This book is dedicated to first about making Wall Pilates accessible but then opening greater possibilities to you. Would I love for you to graduate to 15-minute, or even say, 30-minute intense Pilates workouts? Absolutely. However, for now, I figure we just settle onto those proverbial training wheels and step into how the Weekly Plans work.

The Weekly Plans: Up to 5-minutes exercises, done just once a day

The Weekly Plans covered after this give you that right mix-and-match for a balanced routine. What's great is it allows you to easily level-up when you think you are ready for the next skill level. Here's a quick run-through:

1. **Pick Your Skill Level:** If you're just starting out in this journey

of Pilates, start with "Beginner Weekly Plan". If you are somewhat experienced with Pilates, go to "Intermediate Weekly Plan". If "Beginner" and "Intermediate" are clearly not your speed or you are progressing fast, hit up the "Advanced Weekly Plan".

2. **Select the day of the week:** The schedule is divided up by days of the week - Monday, Tuesday, Wednesday, Thursday, Friday, Saturday (minus Sunday as rest day). You can change that up as you need, the weekly plan is just there to make it more convenient. The plan doesn't vary from week-to-week, but that's intentional. It keeps it simpler and pushes you to progress. As you adhere to the weekly plan, you will progress from Beginner to Intermediate and then eventually from Intermediate to Advanced and finally from Advanced to higher intensity workouts.

3. **Follow the 5-minute exercise or as much as you can do:** The workouts start with stretching and lower-intensity exercises, changing what you are doing each day. In the weekly plan, the illustrated exercise with instruction on how to perform said exercise is added for your convenience. With time, you will familiarize yourself with each exercise and be able to perform the workout with ease. Challenge yourself to complete all 5 minutes - but again, if find that you only have just that 1-minute, work first on the lower intensity exercises. However, if you are already feeling limber for that day, attempt one of the higher intensity exercises.

Are you limited to up to 5-minutes?

Not by a long shot. You can double-down to 10-minutes or even triple-down your time to 15-minutes using the workouts from this book. The sky is the limit. You have my full blessing to mix it up and try new things or just keep doing what works for you by repeating the same workouts you know and love.

Wall Pilates isn't just about getting in shape; it's about fitting fitness seamlessly into your life. With this guide, you're not just doing exercises; you're unlocking a new way to live healthily, no matter how packed your schedule is. So, welcome to the world of Wall Pilates – where every minute is an opportunity, and every effort brings you closer to your best self. Let's do this!

II

Beginner Weekly Plan

This plan is for a 5-minute exercise routine for days Monday through Saturday, tailored to fit a variety of focus areas and intensity levels, ensuring a well-rounded workout experience throughout the week.

You got this – no excuses!

Please remember to BREATHE during and between each exercise.

Beginner Monday

- **1st Minute:** Beginner - Core/Abs - **Wall Plank**
- **2nd Minute:** Beginner - Core/Abs - **Wall Mountain Climbers**
- **3rd Minute:** Beginner - Core/Abs - **Standing Wall Roll-Down**
- **4th Minute:** Beginner - Balance/Stability - **Wall Tree Pose**
- **5th Minute**: Beginner - Balance/Stability - **Wall Warrior II**

See Illustrations and How to Perform Exercise below

* * *

1st Minute: Beginner - Core/Abs - Wall Plank

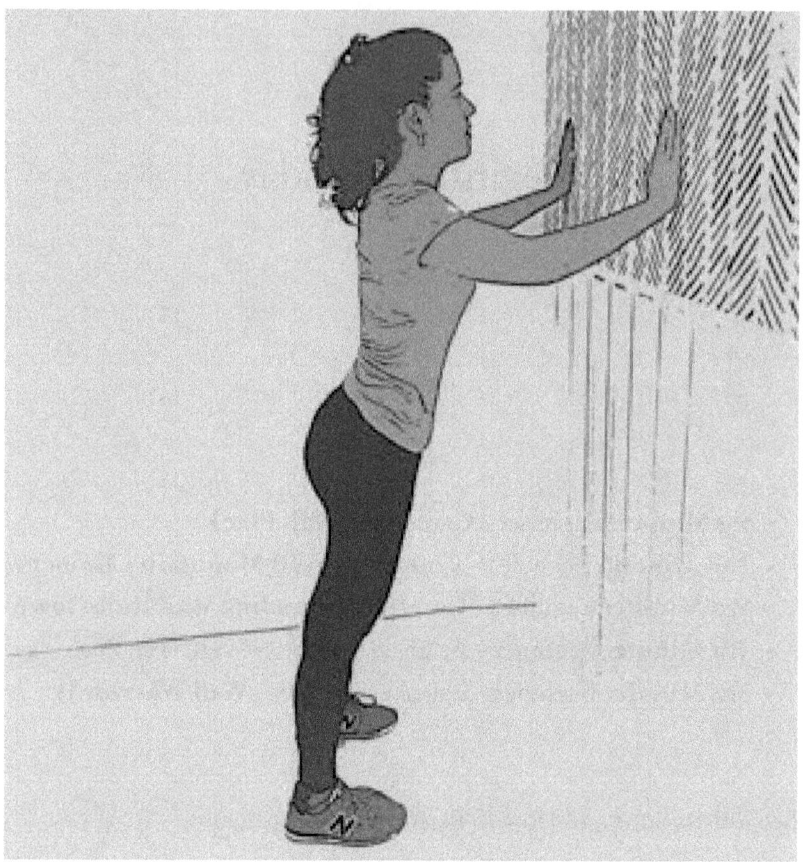

Wall Plank: Stand facing the wall, place hands on the wall at shoulder height, step back until body is in a straight line from head to heels, engage your core.

* * *

2nd Minute: Beginner - Core/Abs - Wall Mountain Climbers

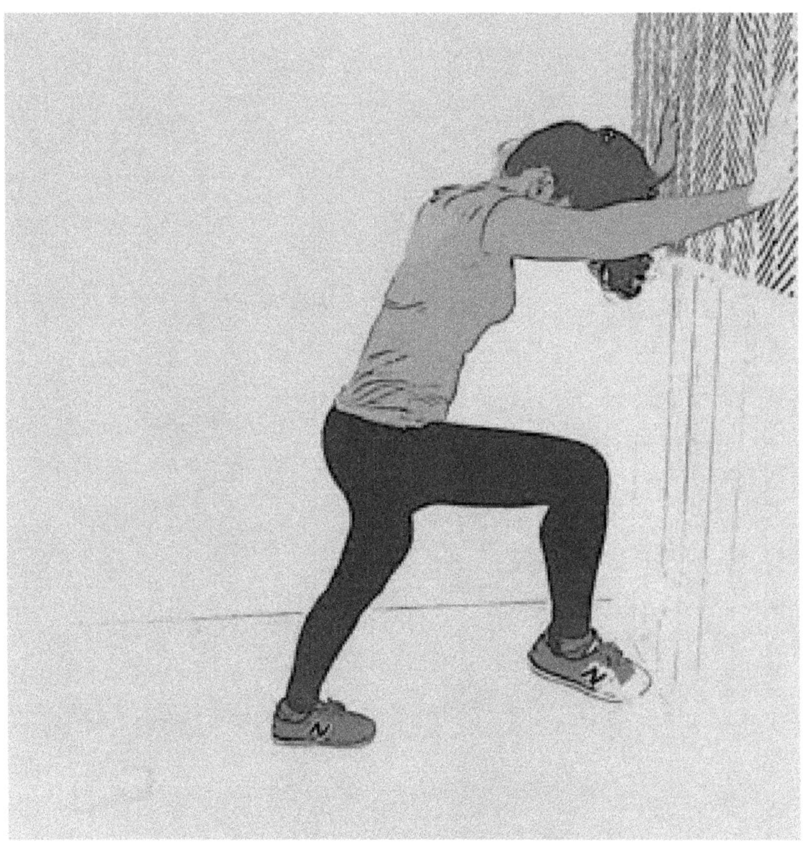

Wall Mountain Climbers: Stand facing the wall, place hands on the wall at shoulder height, alternate driving your knees up towards your chest in a controlled manner.

* * *

3rd Minute: Beginner - Core/Abs - Standing Wall Roll-Down

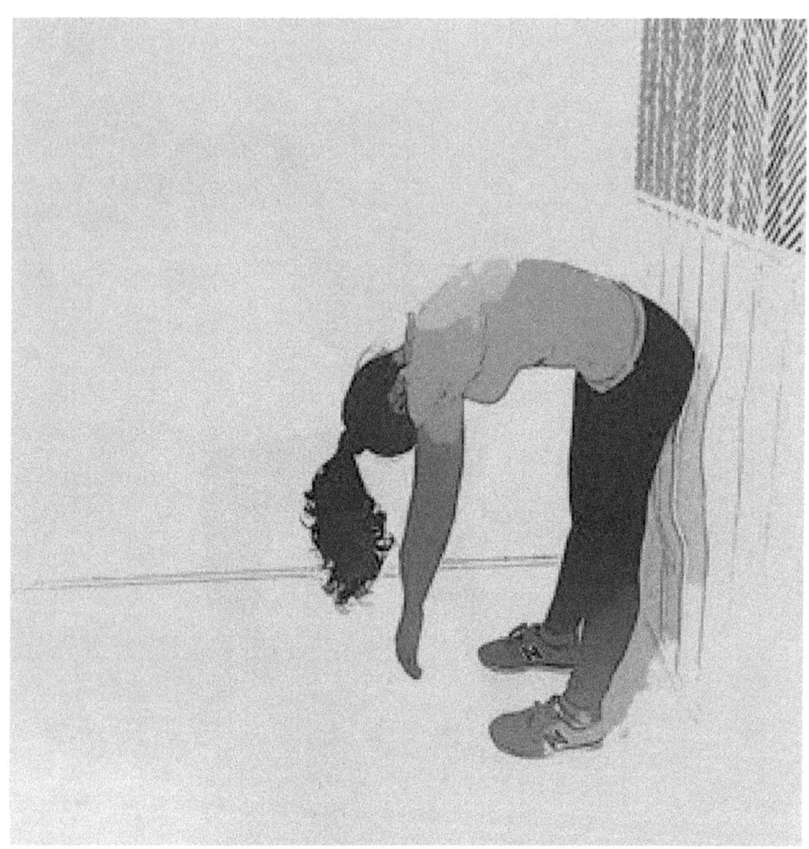

Standing Wall Roll-Down: Stand with your back to the wall, slowly roll down vertebra by vertebra until hands touch the ground. Alternatively, walk hands down the wall until body is parallel to the floor, then once they touch, walk them back up.

* * *

4th Minute: Beginner - Balance/Stability - Wall Tree Pose

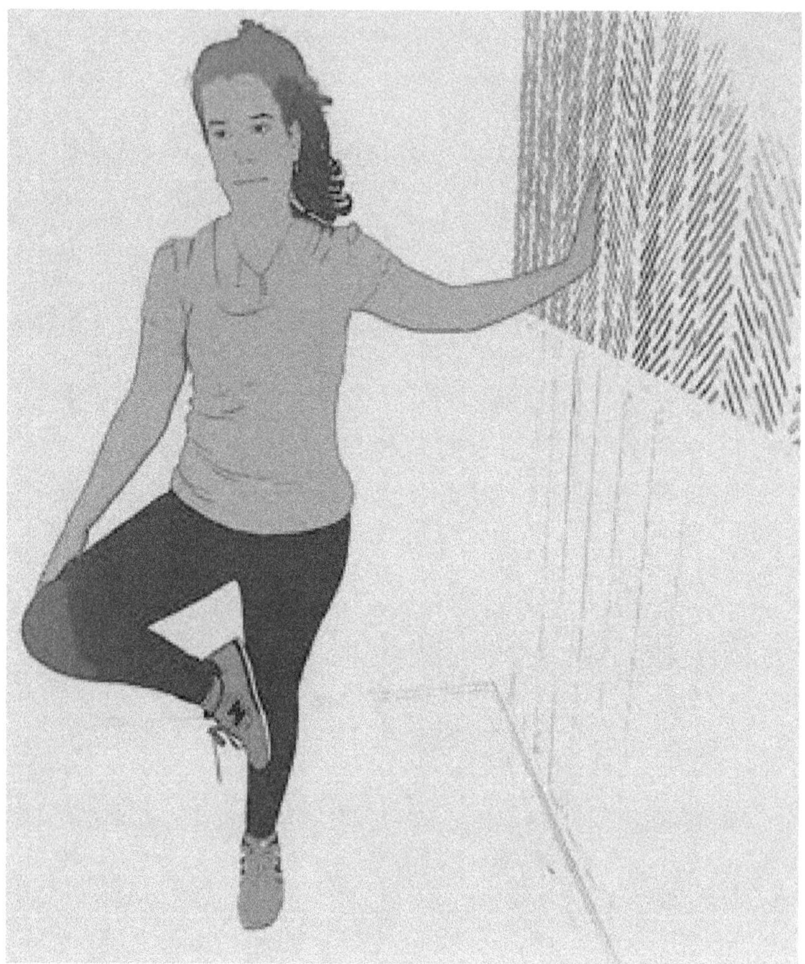

Wall Tree Pose: Stand with side to wall, place foot of one leg on inner thigh of the other, use wall for balance. For advanced, raise hands over head to simulate a "Tree Pose".

* * *

5th Minute: Beginner - Balance/Stability - Wall Warrior II

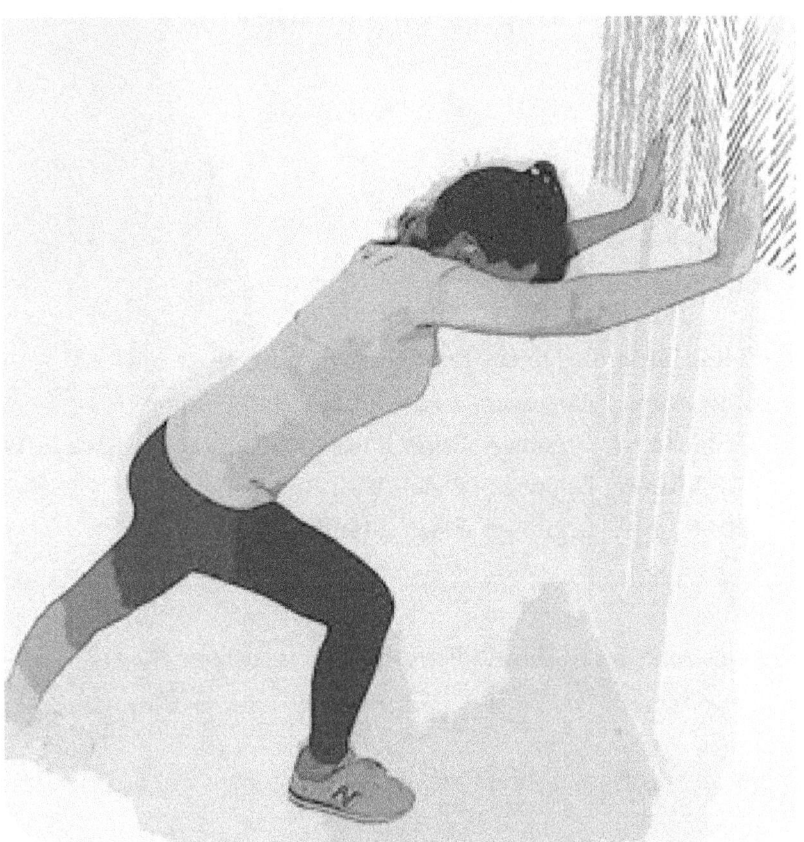

Wall Warrior II: Stand facing the wall, lean forward with hands on the wall, plant one leg far back at 45 degree angle, keep body and extended leg in a straight line.

Beginner Tuesday

- **1st Minute**: Beginner - Legs/Glutes - **Wall Squat**
- **2nd Minute**: Beginner - Legs/Glutes - **Wall Bridges**
- **3rd Minute**: Beginner - Legs/Glutes - **Wall Squat with Toe Lifts**
- **4th Minute**: Beginner - Back - **Wall Angels**
- **5th Minute**: Beginner - Back - **Standing Wall Press**

See Illustrations and How to Perform Exercise below

* * *

1st Minute: Beginner - Legs/Glutes - Wall Squat

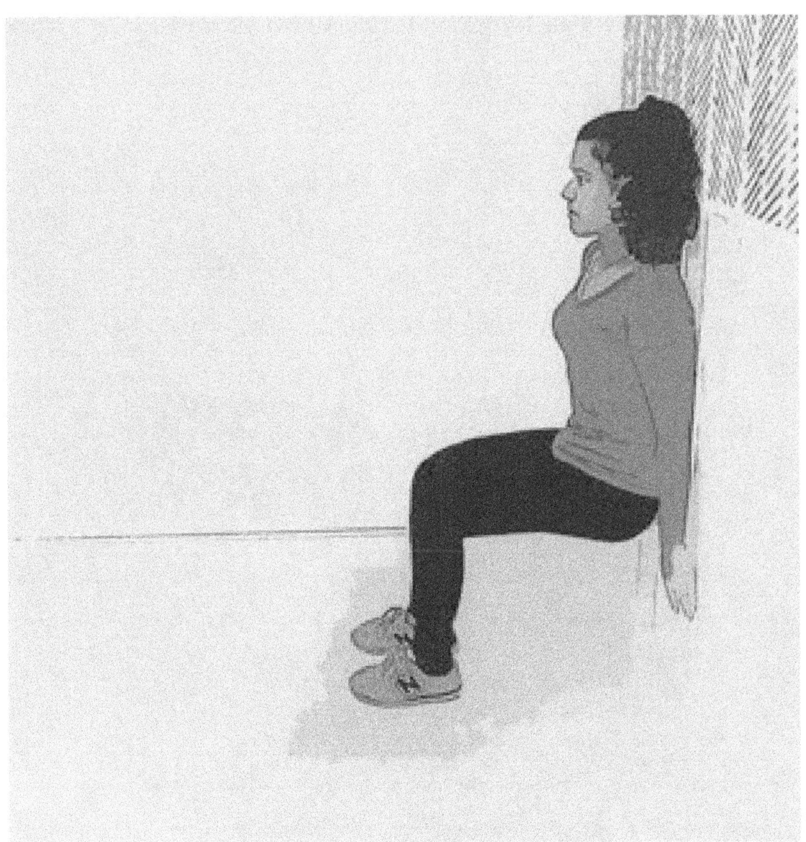

Wall Squat: With back against the wall, lower into a squat until thighs are parallel to the floor, then stand back up.

* * *

2nd Minute: Beginner - Legs/Glutes - Wall Bridges

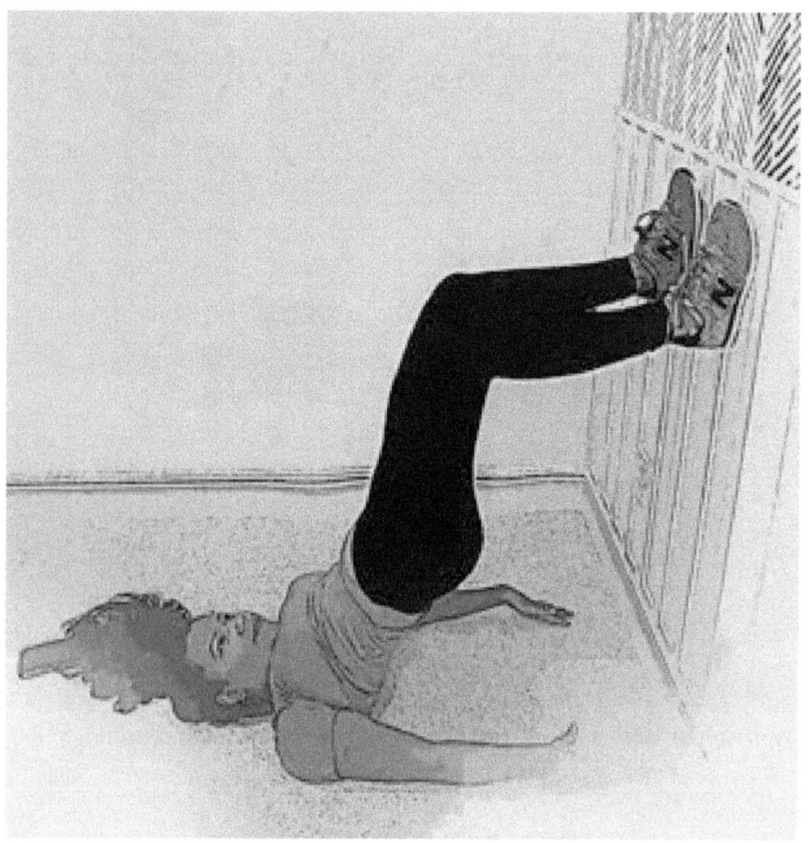

Wall Bridges: Lie on your back with feet flat against the wall, knees bent, lift hips towards the ceiling, then lower them back down.

* * *

3rd Minute: Beginner - Legs/Glutes - Wall Squat with Toe Lifts

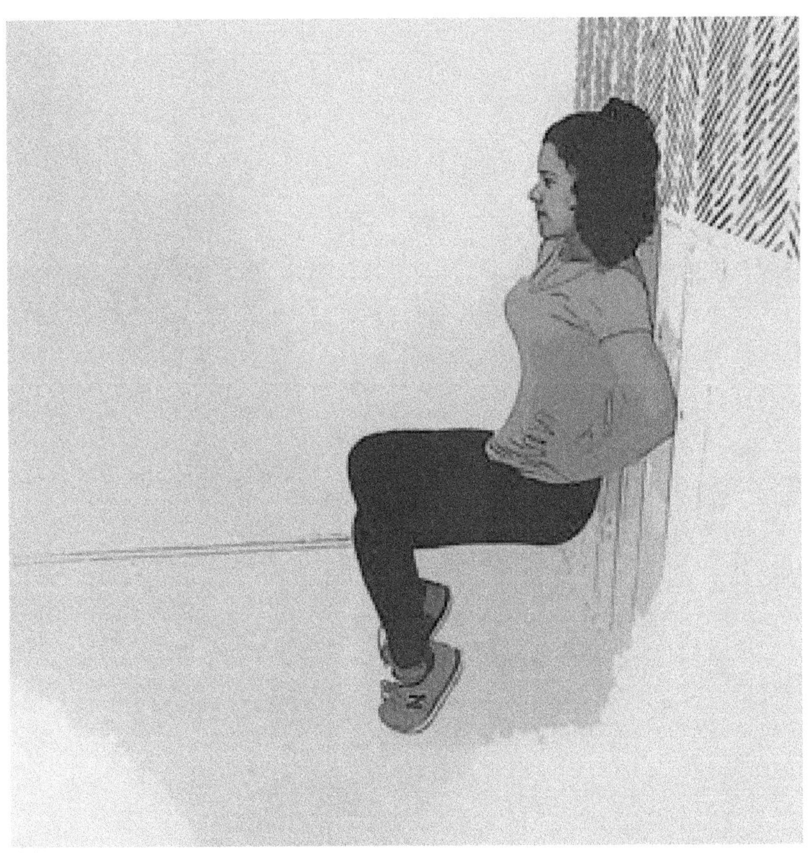

Wall Squats with Toe Lifts: In a wall squat position, lift toes off the ground alternately while maintaining the squat.

* * *

4th Minute: Beginner - Back - Wall Angels

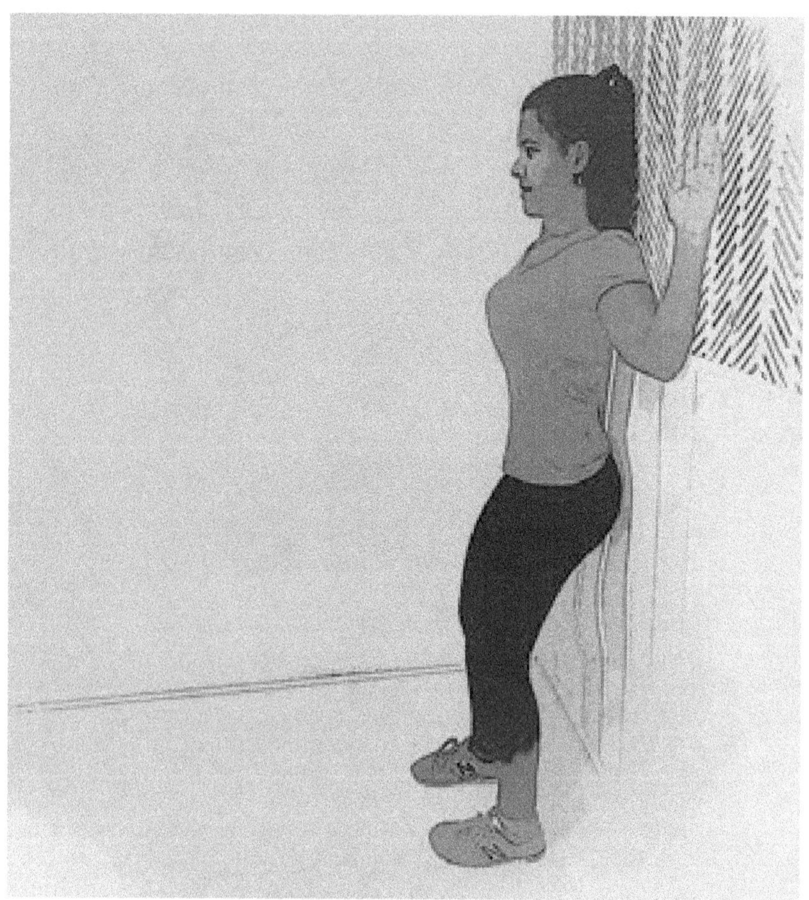

Wall Angels - Part 1: Stand with back against the wall, keep arms held against the wall and point forearm up vertically towards ceiling.

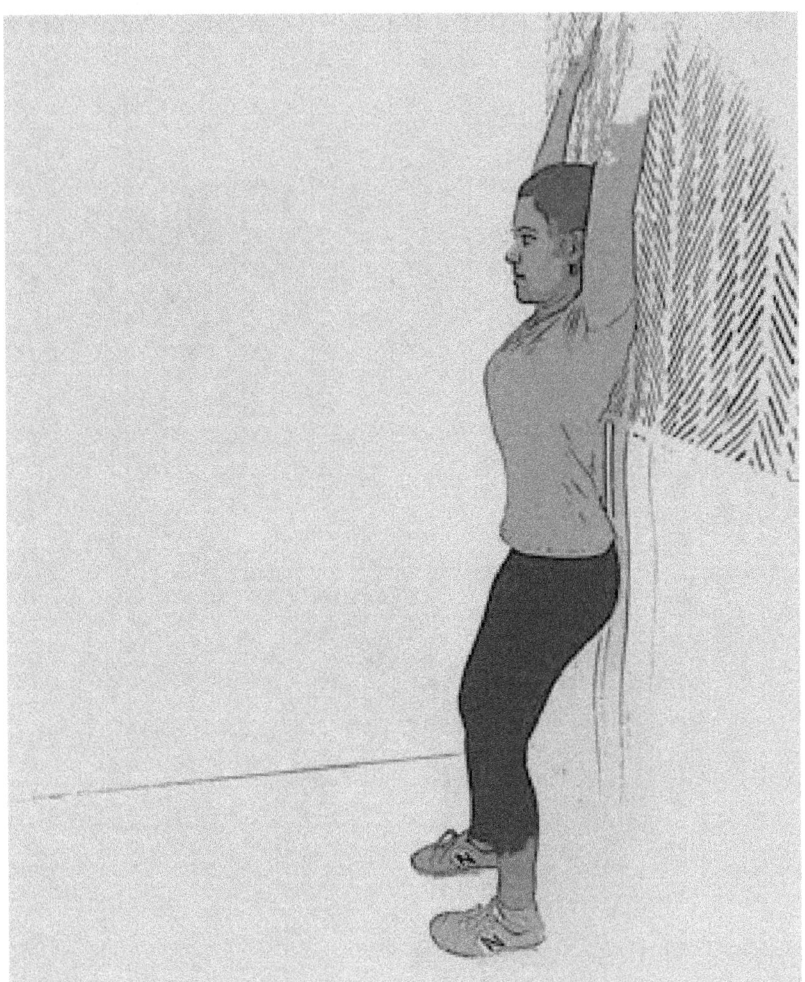

Wall Angels - Part 2: Holding your position against the wall, raise arms up straight while still pressing them against wall. Then bring them back down to the first position and repeat.

* * *

5th Minute: Beginner - Back - Standing Wall Press

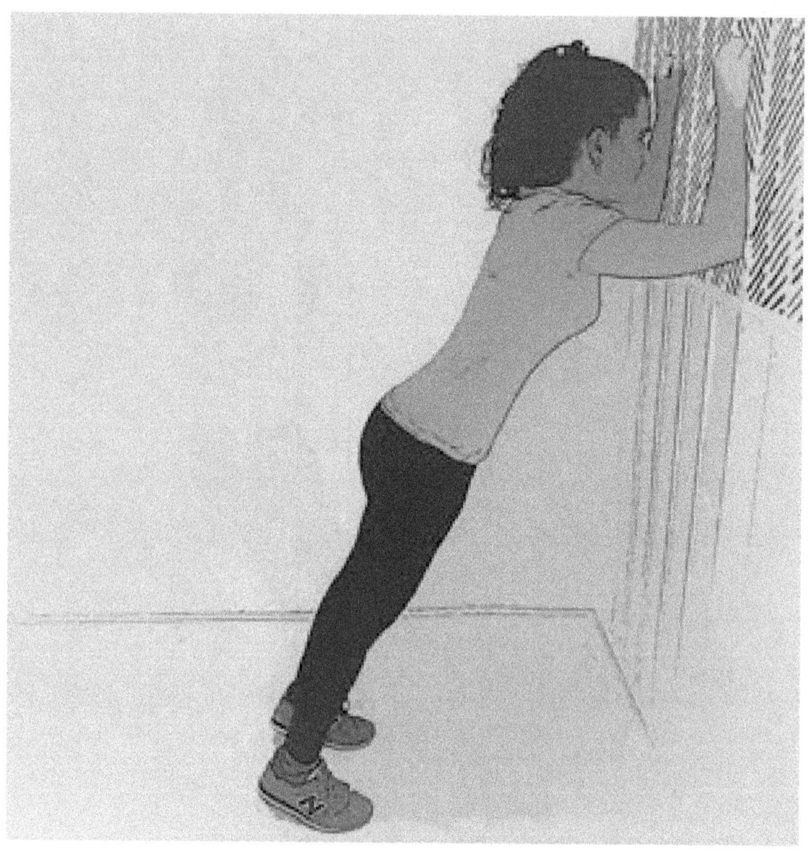

Standing Wall Press: Stand facing the wall, press forearms into the wall at shoulder height as if trying to push the wall away.

Beginner Wednesday

- **1st minute**: Beginner - Upper Body - **Wall Chest Stretch**
- **2nd minute**: Beginner - Upper Body - **Wall Push-Ups**
- **3rd minute**: Beginner - Upper Body - **Standing Wall Press**
- **4th minute**: Beginner - Flexibility/Mobility - **Wall Hamstring Stretch**
- **5th minute**: Beginner - Flexibility/Mobility - **Wall Calf Stretch**

See Illustrations and How to Perform Exercise below

* * *

1st minute: Beginner - Upper Body - Wall Chest Stretch

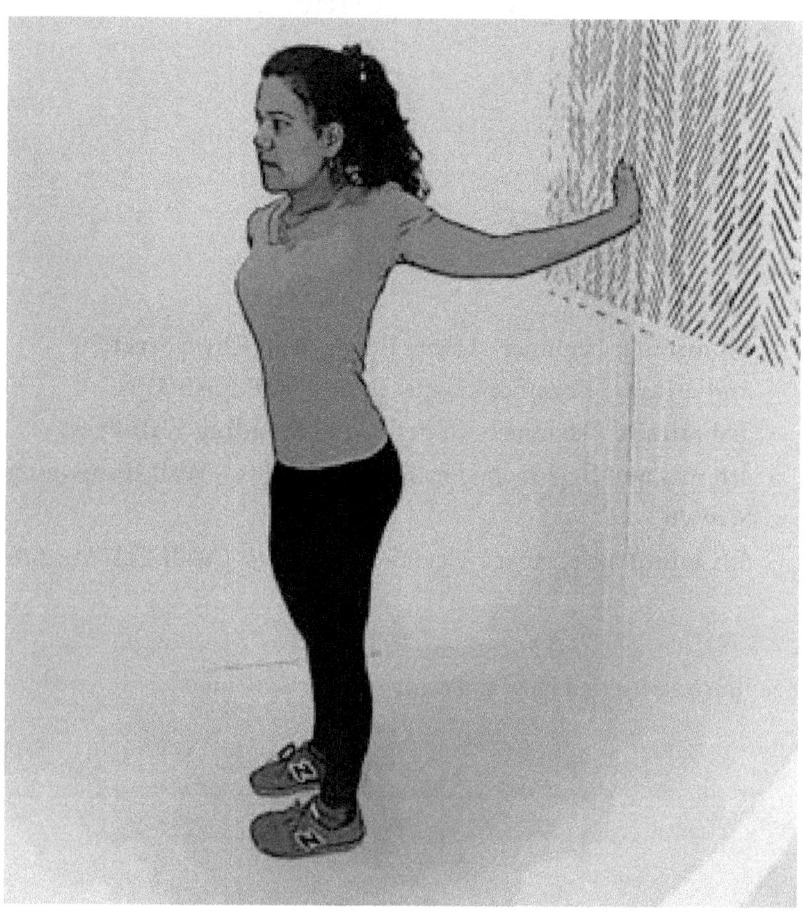

Wall Chest Stretch: Face away from the wall, place one hand on it behind you, slowly turn and shift forward until you feel a stretch in your chest and shoulders. Switch arms.

* * *

2nd minute: Beginner - Upper Body - Wall Push-Ups

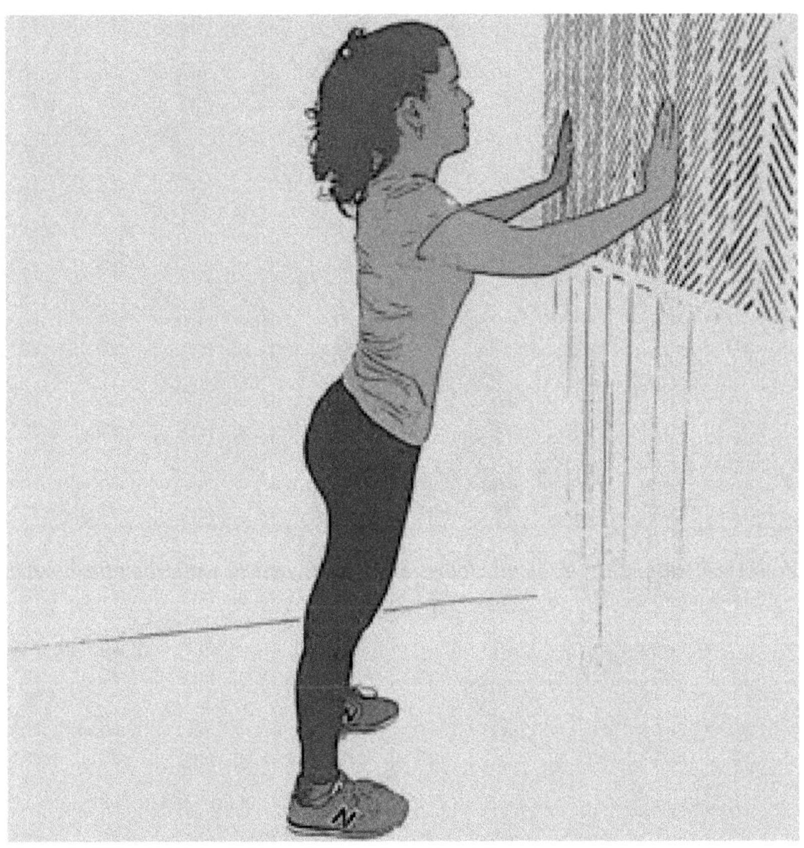

Wall Push-ups - Part 1: Stand facing the wall, place hands on wall in front of you at shoulder width.

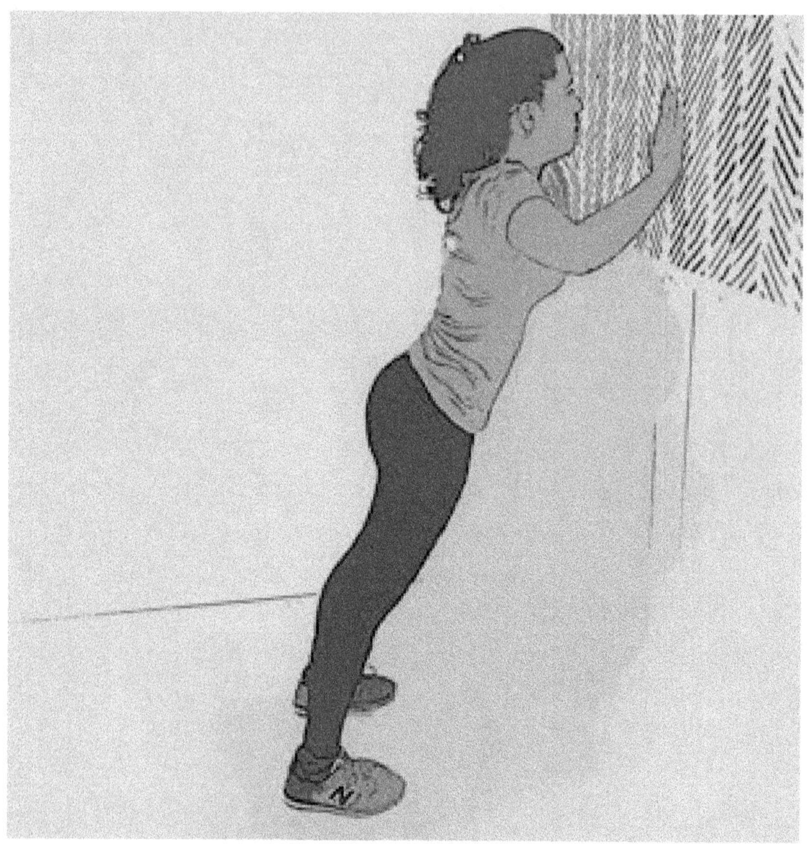

Wall Push-ups - Part 2: Bend elbows and lower chest to wall, then push back. Repeat.

* * *

3rd minute: Beginner - Upper Body - Standing Wall Press

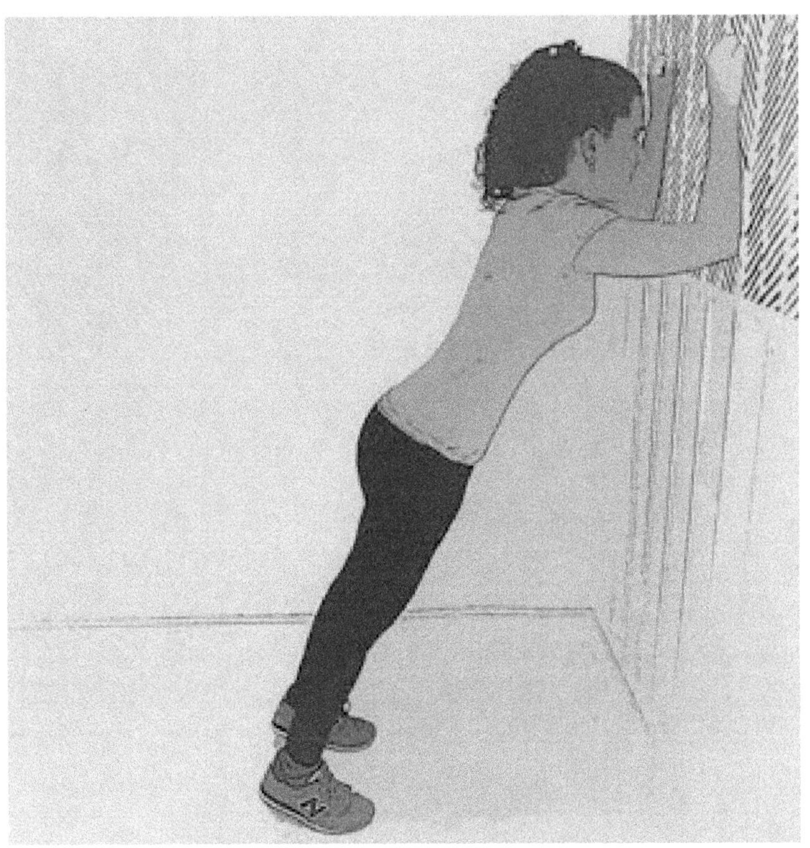

Standing Wall Press: Stand facing the wall, press forearms into the wall at shoulder height as if trying to push the wall away.

* * *

4th minute: Beginner - Flexibility/Mobility - Wall Hamstring Stretch

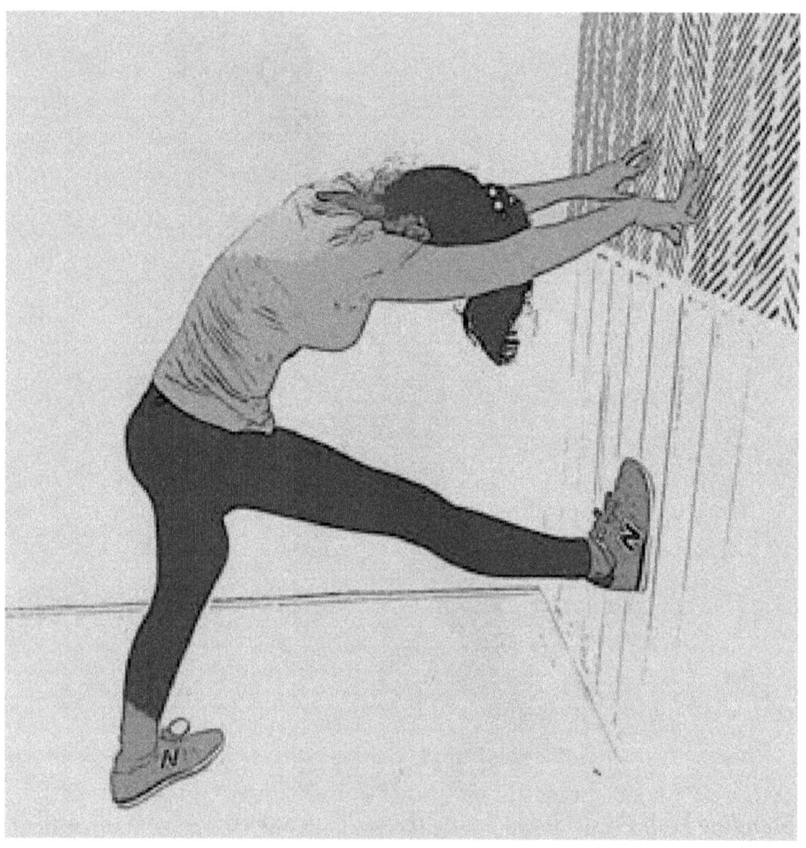

Wall Hamstring Stretch: Place one foot on the wall at hip level, lean forward to stretch the hamstring, switch legs.

* * *

5th minute: Beginner - Flexibility/Mobility - Wall Calf Stretch

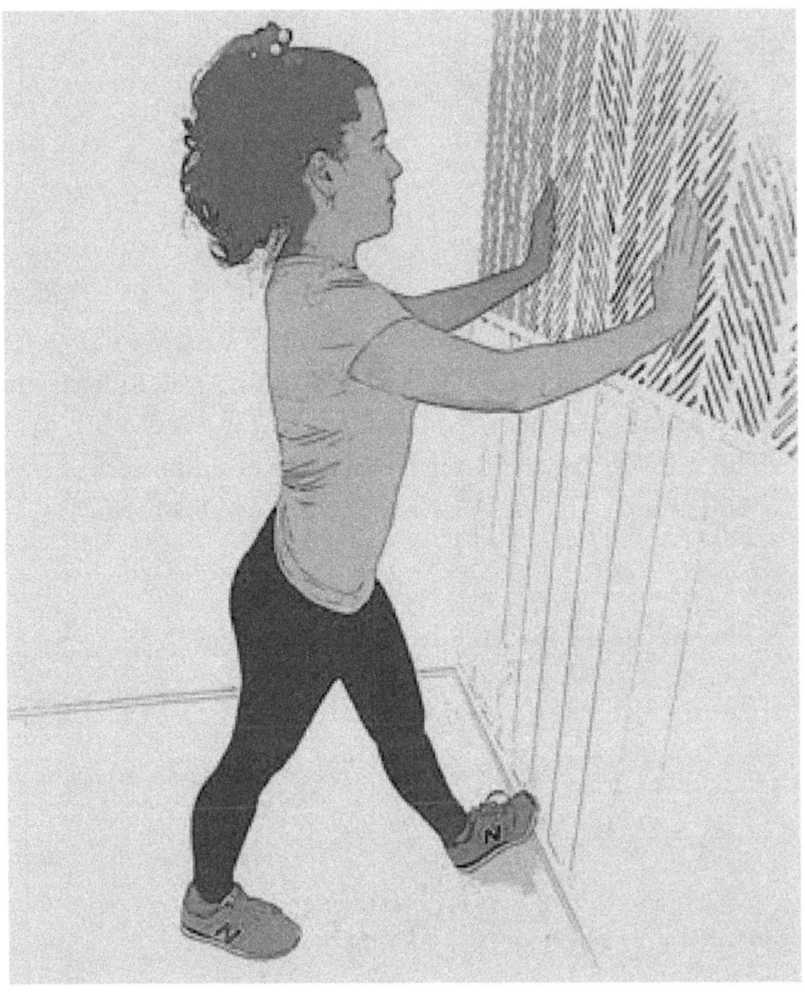

Wall Calf Stretch: Place toes of one foot on the wall, heel on the ground, lean forward to stretch the calf, then switch legs.

Beginner Thursday

- **1st minute**: Beginner - Core/Abs - **Wall Sit with Marching**
- **2nd minute**: Beginner - Core/Abs - **Standing Wall Roll-Down**
- **3rd minute**: Beginner - Full Body Integration - **Wall Walk-Up**
- **4th minute**: Beginner - Balance/Stability - **Wall Butterfly**
- **5th minute**: Beginner - Balance/Stability - **Wall Warrior II**

See Illustrations and How to Perform Exercise below

* * *

1st minute: Beginner - Core/Abs - Wall Sit with Marching

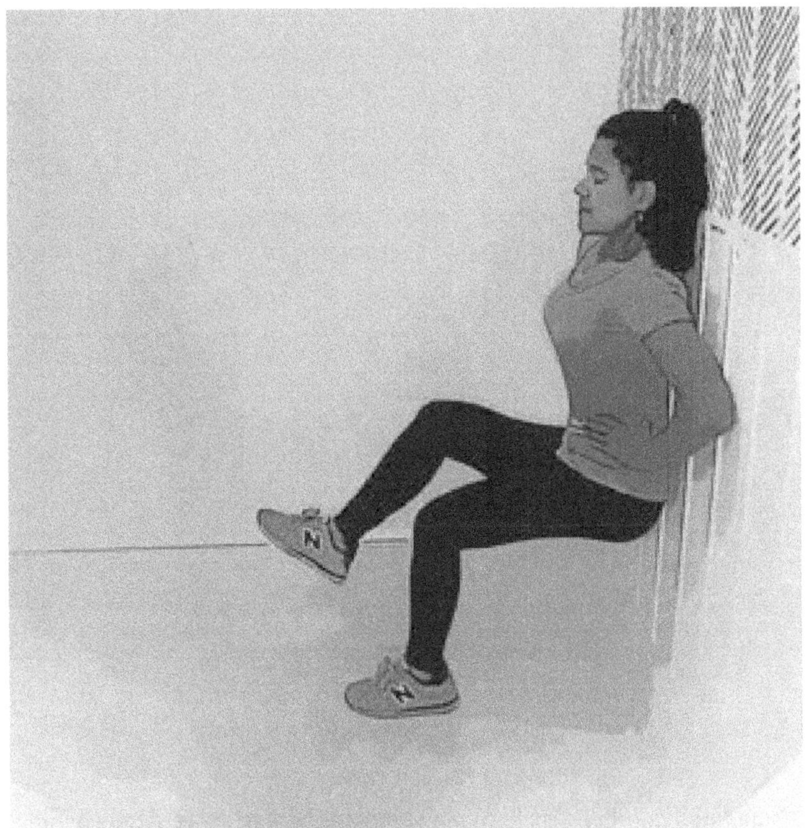

Wall Sit with Marching: Slide down the wall into a sit position with knees at a 90-degree angle, then alternate lifting each knee as if marching.

* * *

2nd minute: Beginner - Core/Abs - Standing Wall Roll-Down

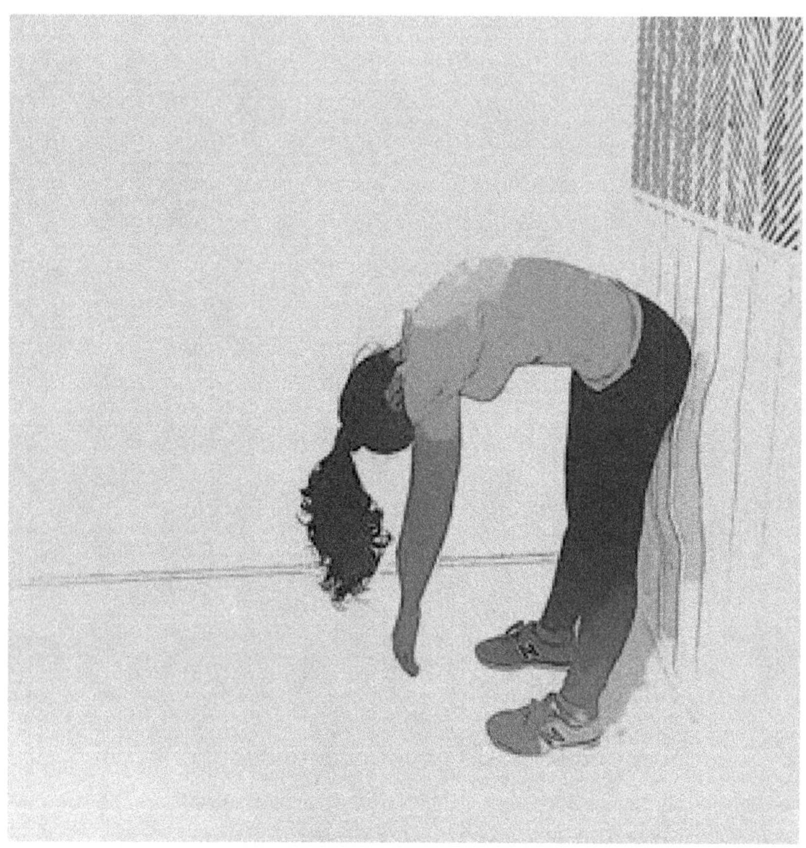

Standing Wall Roll-Down: Stand with your back to the wall, slowly roll down vertebra by vertebra until hands touch the ground. Alternatively, walk hands down the wall until body is parallel to the floor, then once they touch, walk them back up.

* * *

3rd minute: Beginner - Full Body Integration - Wall Walk-Up

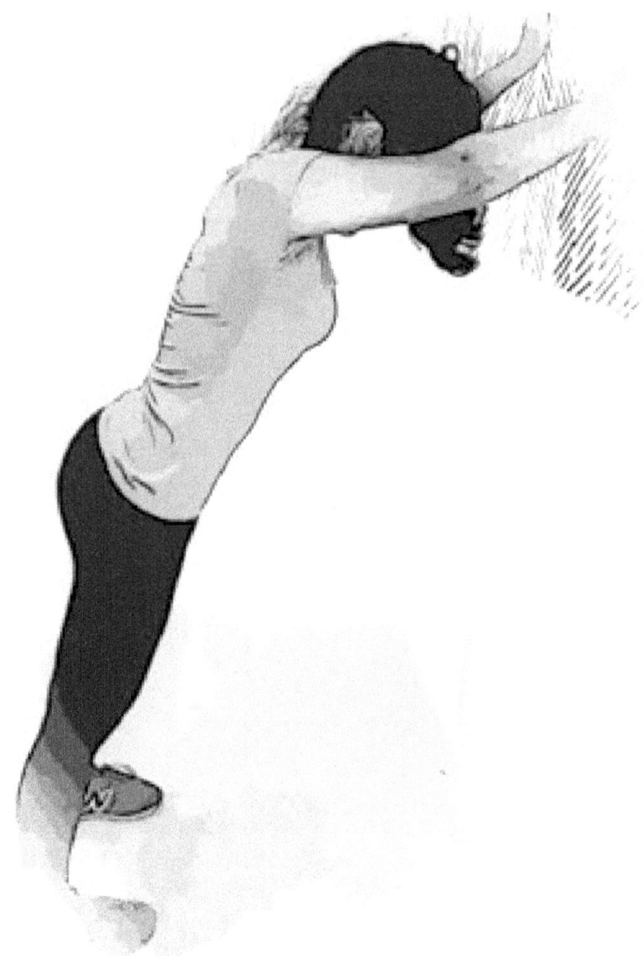

Wall Walk-Up: Face the wall, place hands on it, walk hands up as high as possible, then walk them back down.

* * *

4th minute: Beginner - Balance/Stability - Wall Butterfly

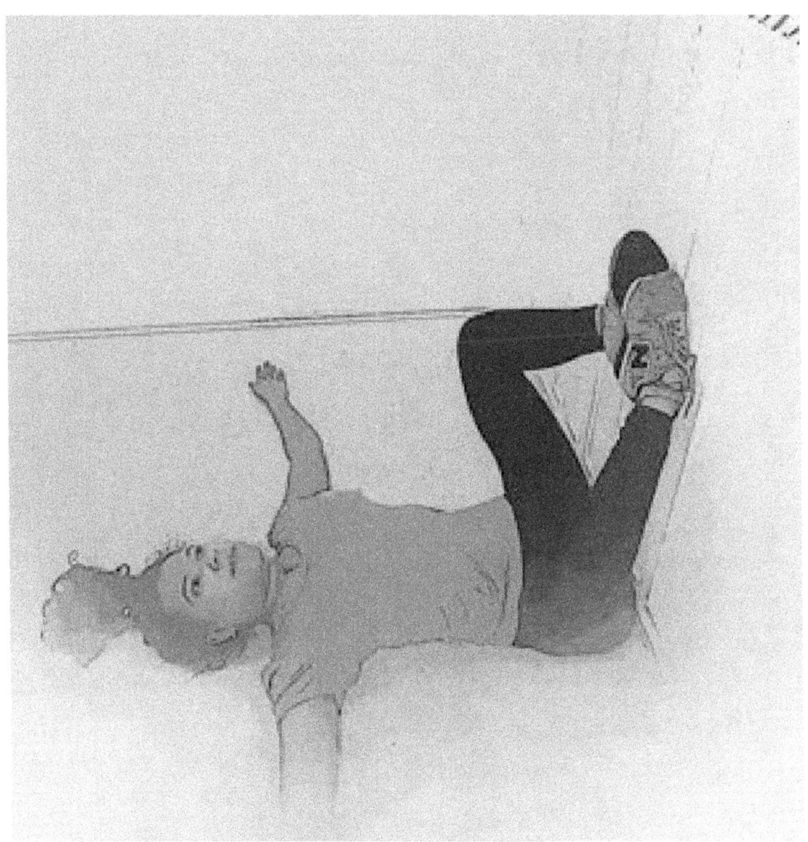

Wall Butterfly: Sit with back against the floor, soles of feet together, knees open to sides, press knees gently in towards wall. Alternatively, for a modified version, sit with back against the wall, soles of feet together, knees open to sides, press knees gently towards floor.

* * *

5th minute: Beginner - Balance/Stability - Wall Warrior II

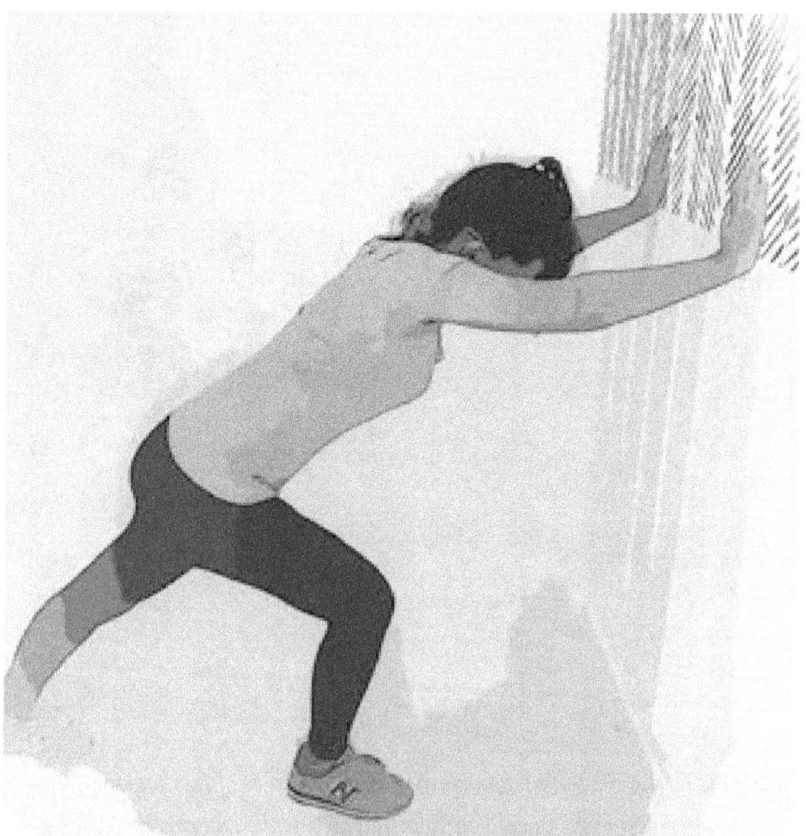

Wall Warrior II: Stand facing the wall, lean forward with hands on the wall, plant one leg far back at 45 degree angle, keep body and extended leg in a straight line.

Beginner Friday

- **1st minute**: Beginner - Legs/Glutes - **Wall Side Leg Lifts**
- **2nd minute**: Beginner - Legs/Glutes - **Wall Squat with Toe Lifts**
- **3rd minute**: Beginner - Full Body Integration - **Wall Arm Circle With One Arm**
- **4th minute**: Beginner - Back - **Wall Angels**
- **5th minute**: Beginner - Back - **Standing Wall Press**

See Illustrations and How to Perform Exercise below

* * *

1st minute: Beginner - Legs/Glutes - Wall Side Leg Lifts

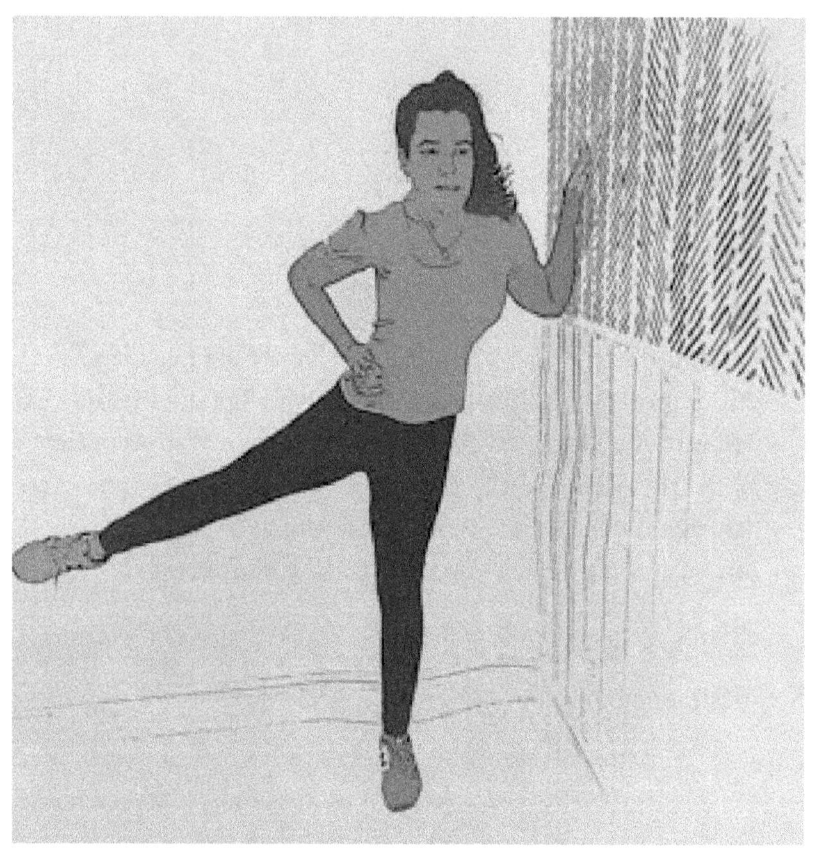

Wall Side Leg Lifts: Stand with your side to the wall for support, lift leg sideways away from body, then lower back down.

* * *

2nd minute: Beginner - Legs/Glutes - Wall Squat with Toe Lifts

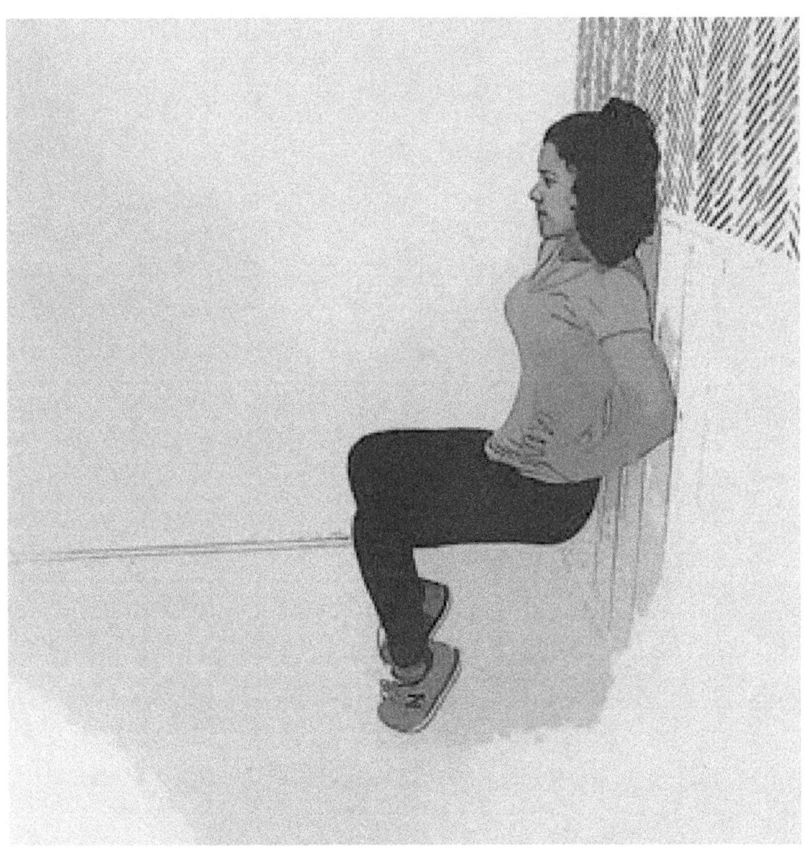

Wall Squats with Toe Lifts: In a wall squat position, lift toes off the ground alternately while maintaining the squat.

* * *

3rd minute: Beginner - Full Body Integration - Wall Arm Circle With One Arm

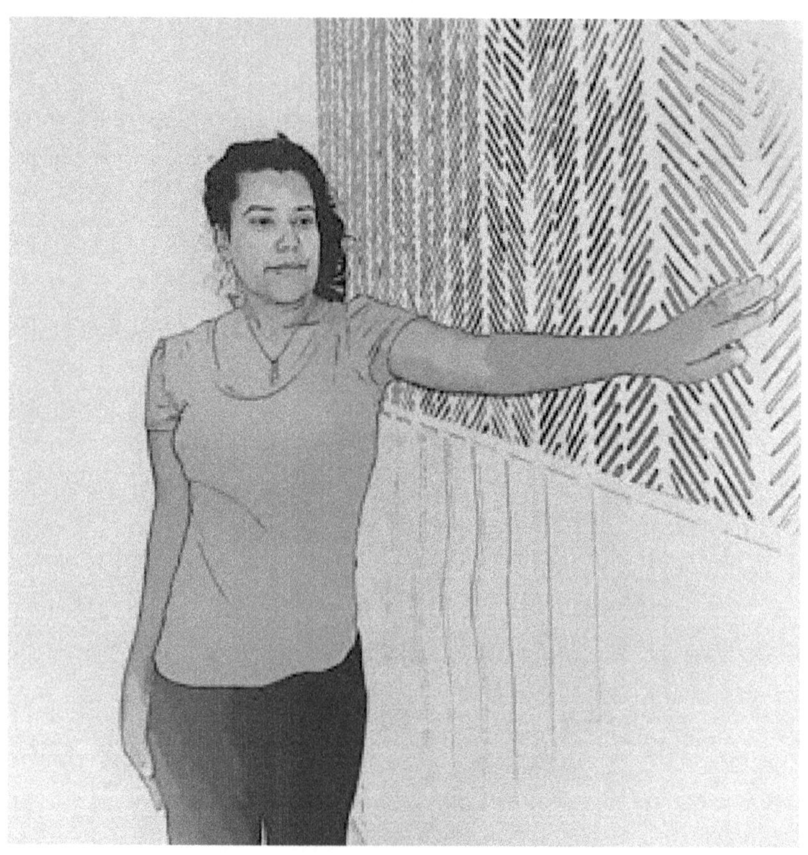

Wall Arm Circle With One Arm - Part 1: Stand straight up and right next to wall, facing the adjacent wall. Extend arm out along the wall.

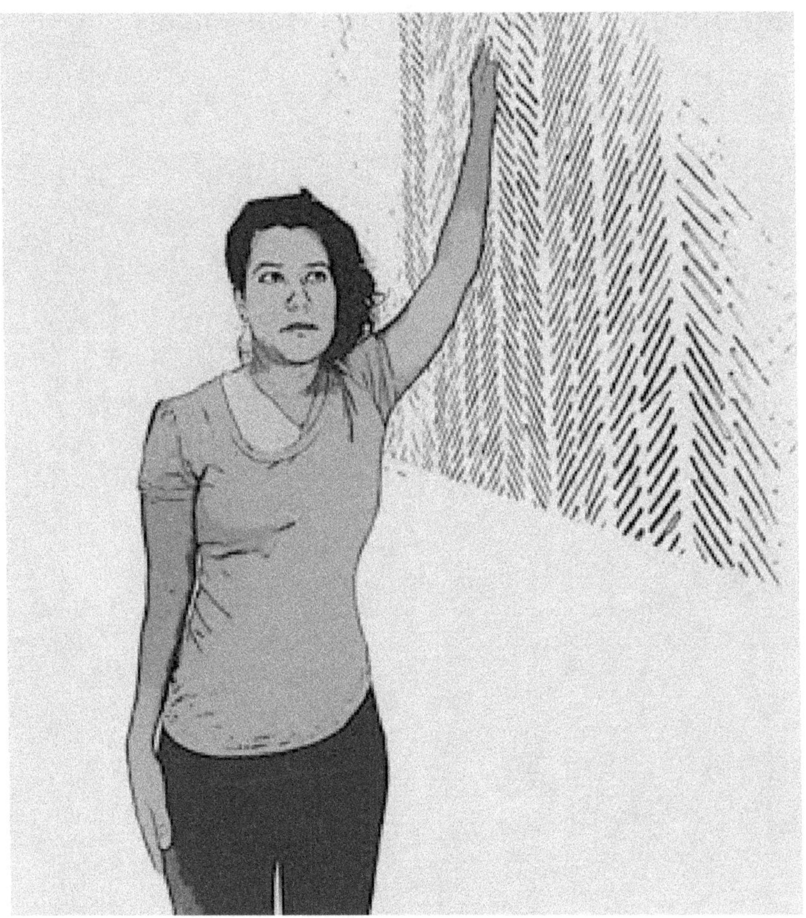

Wall Arm Circle With One Arm - Part 2: Draw a large arms-length circle on the wall around your body as pivot point. Think of your arm as the long arm on a wall clock.

* * *

4th minute: Beginner - Back - Wall Angels

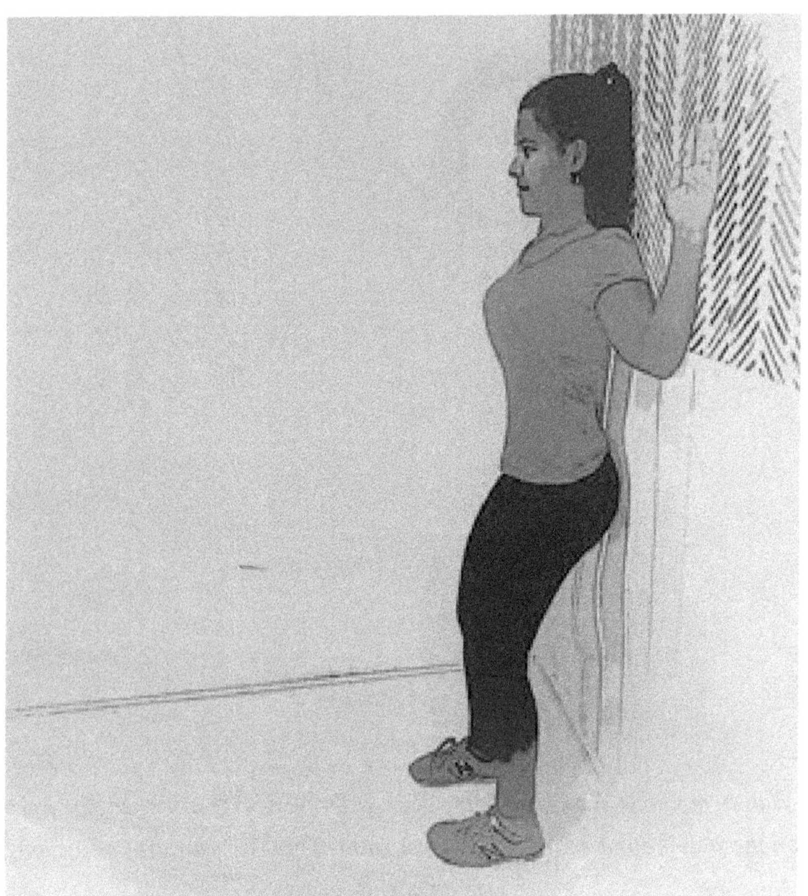

Wall Angels - Part 1: Stand with back against the wall, keep arms held against the wall and point forearm up vertically towards ceiling.

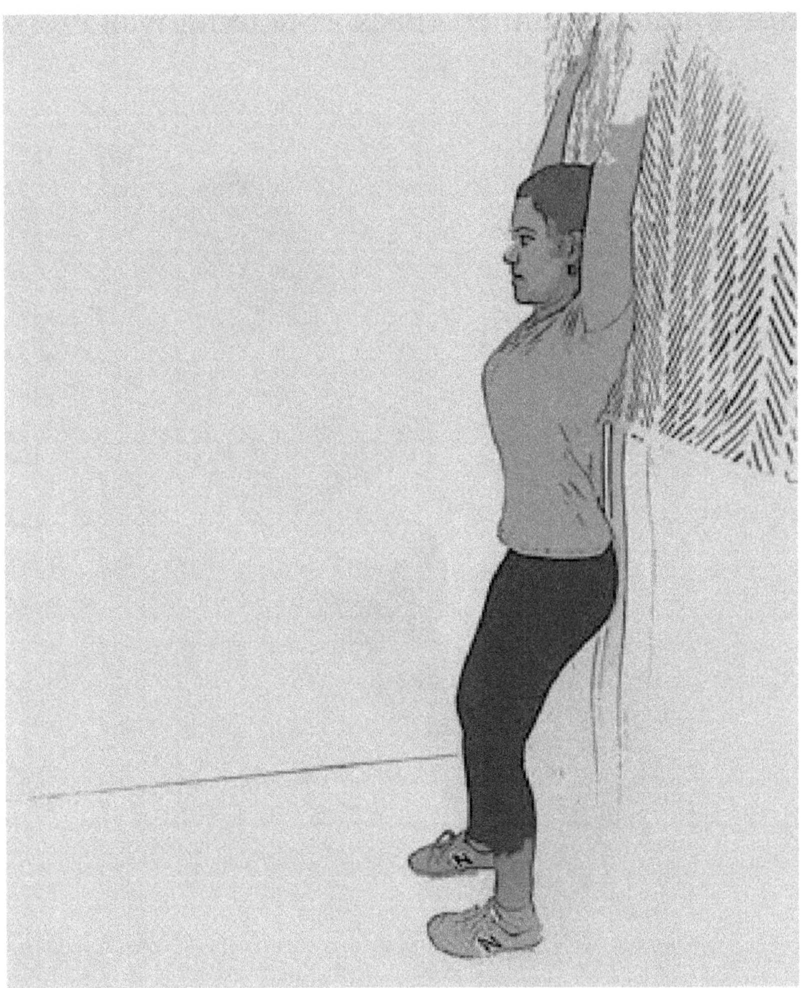

Wall Angels - Part 2: Holding your position against the wall, raise arms up straight while still pressing them against wall. Then bring them back down to the first position and repeat.

* * *

5th minute: Beginner - Back - Standing Wall Press

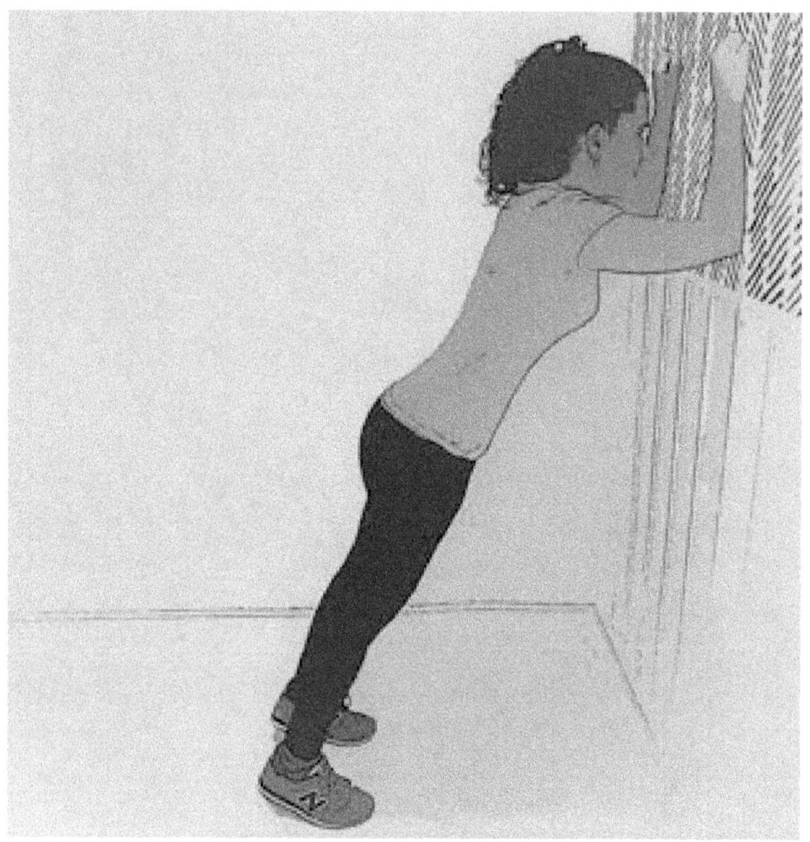

Standing Wall Press: Stand facing the wall, press forearms into the wall at shoulder height as if trying to push the wall away.

Beginner Saturday

- **1st minute**: Beginner - Upper Body - **Wall Tricep Dip Sit Pulses**
- **2nd minute**: Beginner - Upper Body - **Wall Push-Ups**
- **3rd minute**: Beginner - Full Body Integration - **Wall Arm Circle with One Arm**
- **4th minute**: Beginner - Flexibility/Mobility - **Side Bend**
- **5th minute**: Beginner - Flexibility/Mobility - **Reclined Wall Leg Stretch**

See Illustrations and How to Perform Exercise below

* * *

1st minute: Beginner - Upper Body - Wall Tricep Dip Sit Pulses

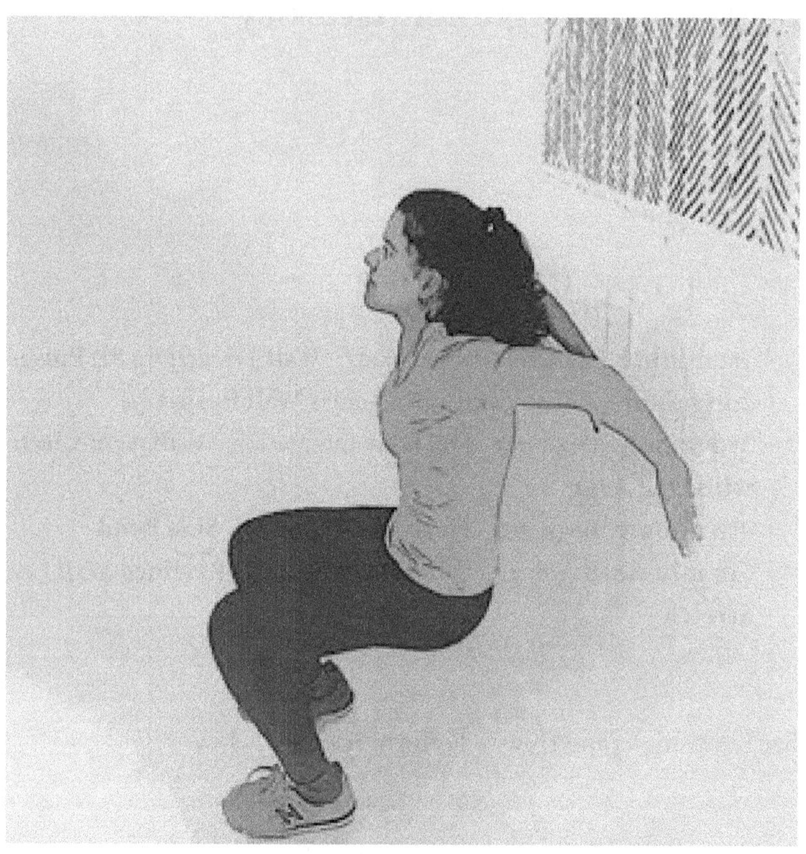

Wall Tricep Dip Sit Pulses: Place hands behind you on wall, lower body by bending elbows, then push back up.

* * *

2nd minute: Beginner - Upper Body - Wall Push-Ups

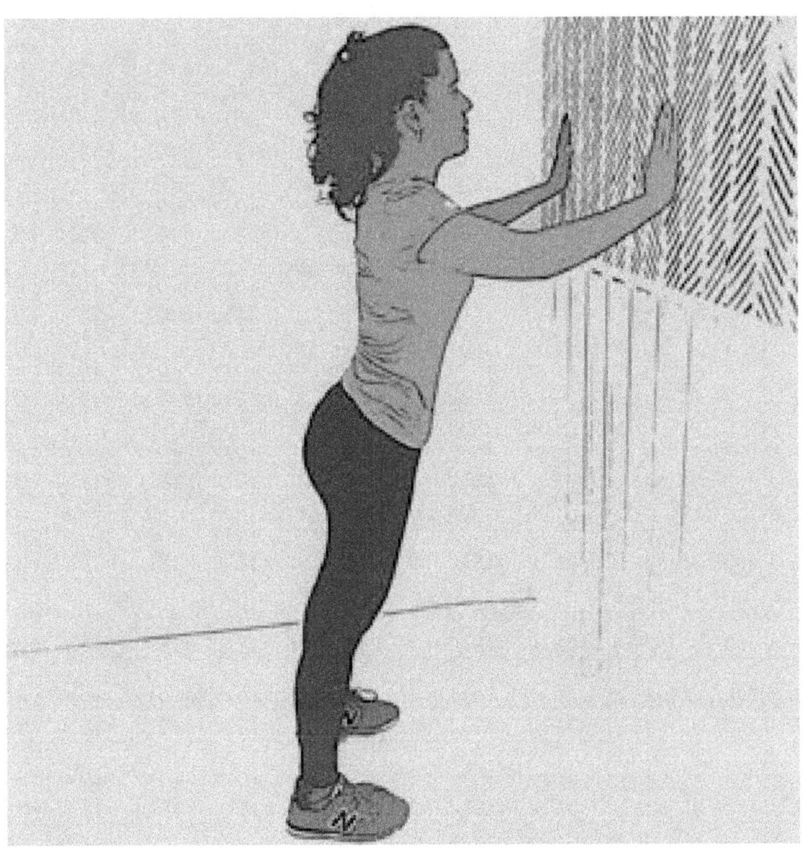

Wall Push-ups - Part 1: Stand facing the wall, place hands on wall in front of you at shoulder width.

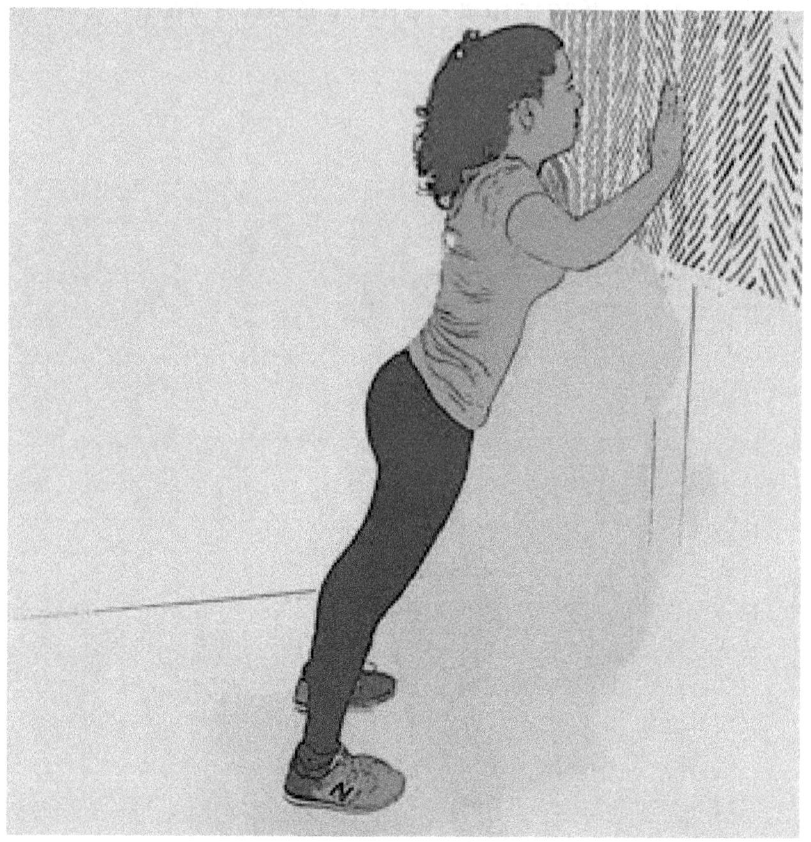

Wall Push-ups - Part 2: Bend elbows and lower chest to wall, then push back. Repeat.

* * *

3rd minute: Beginner - Full Body Integration - Wall Arm Circle with One Arm

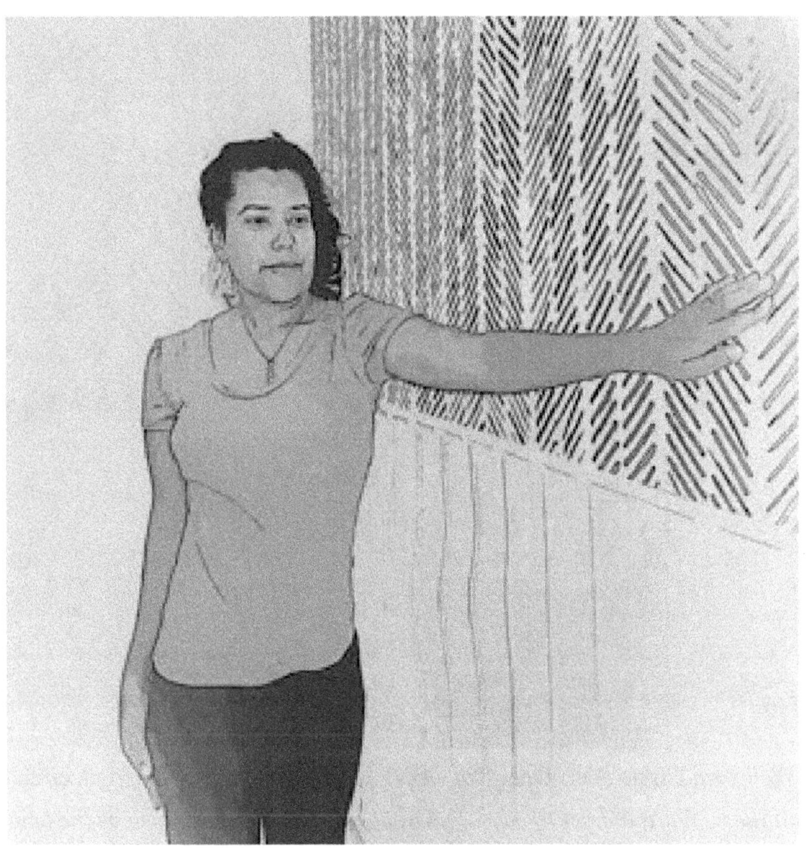

Wall Arm Circle With One Arm - Part 1: Stand straight up and right next to wall, facing the adjacent wall. Extend arm out along the wall.

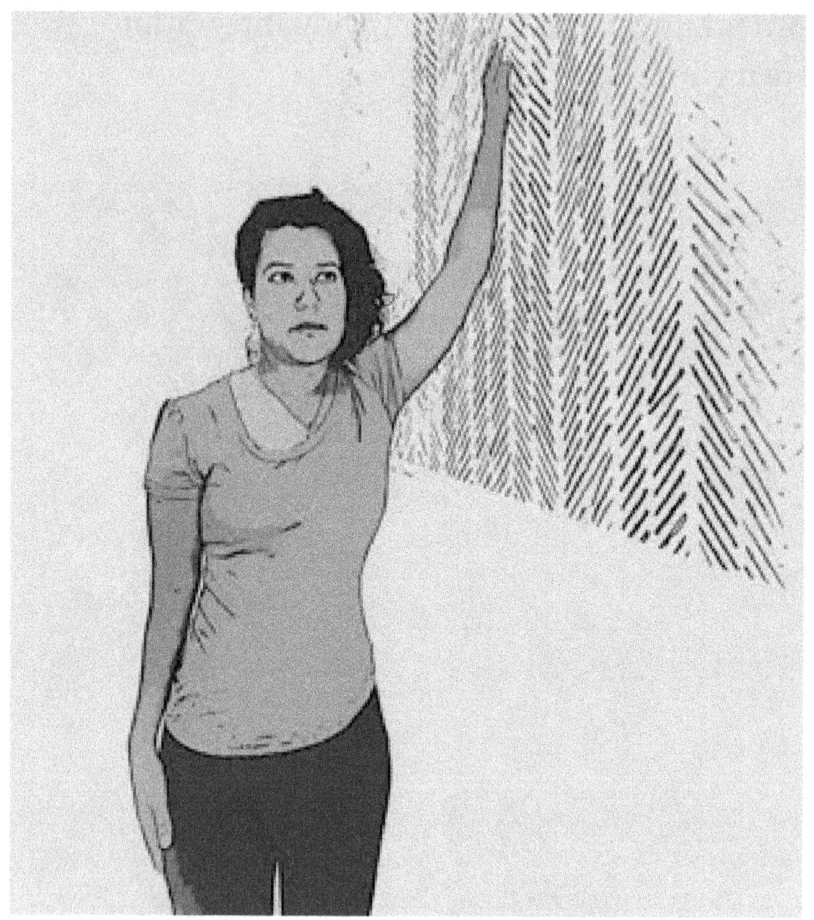

Wall Arm Circle With One Arm - Part 2: Draw a large arms-length circle on the wall around your body as pivot point. Think of your arm as the long arm on a wall clock.

* * *

4th minute: Beginner - Flexibility/Mobility - Side Bend

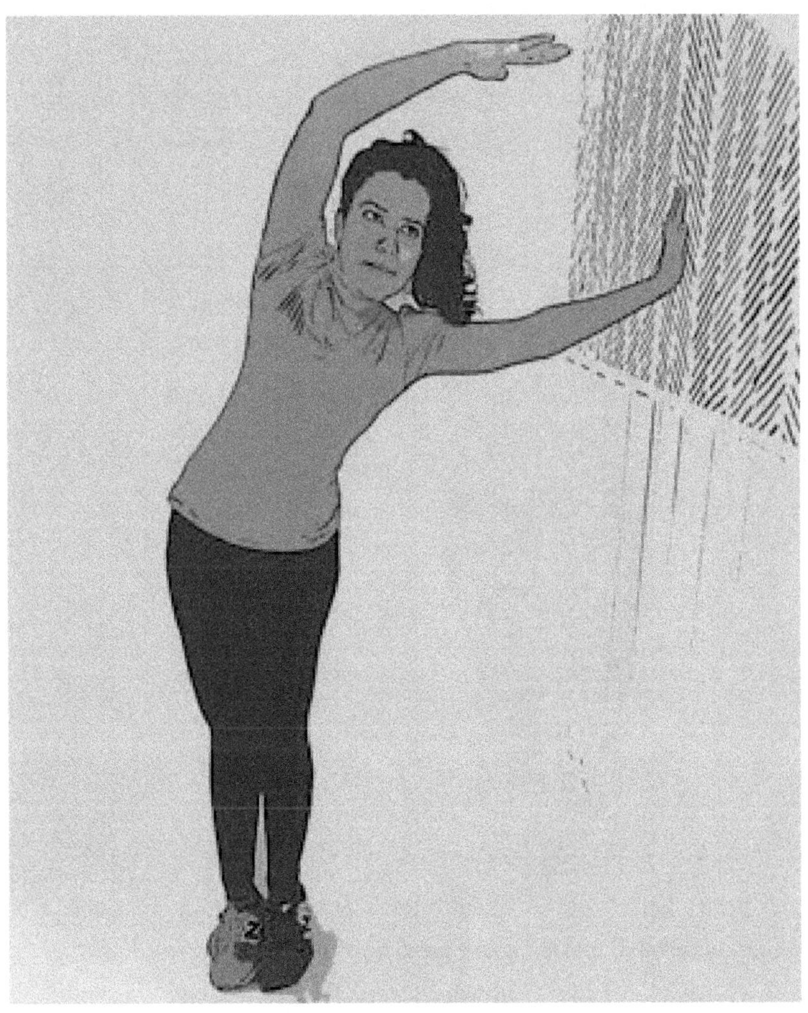

Side Bend - Front View: Stand with left side facing the wall, raise right arm and place hand on wall above head, lean into wall while pushing hips outward, switch sides.

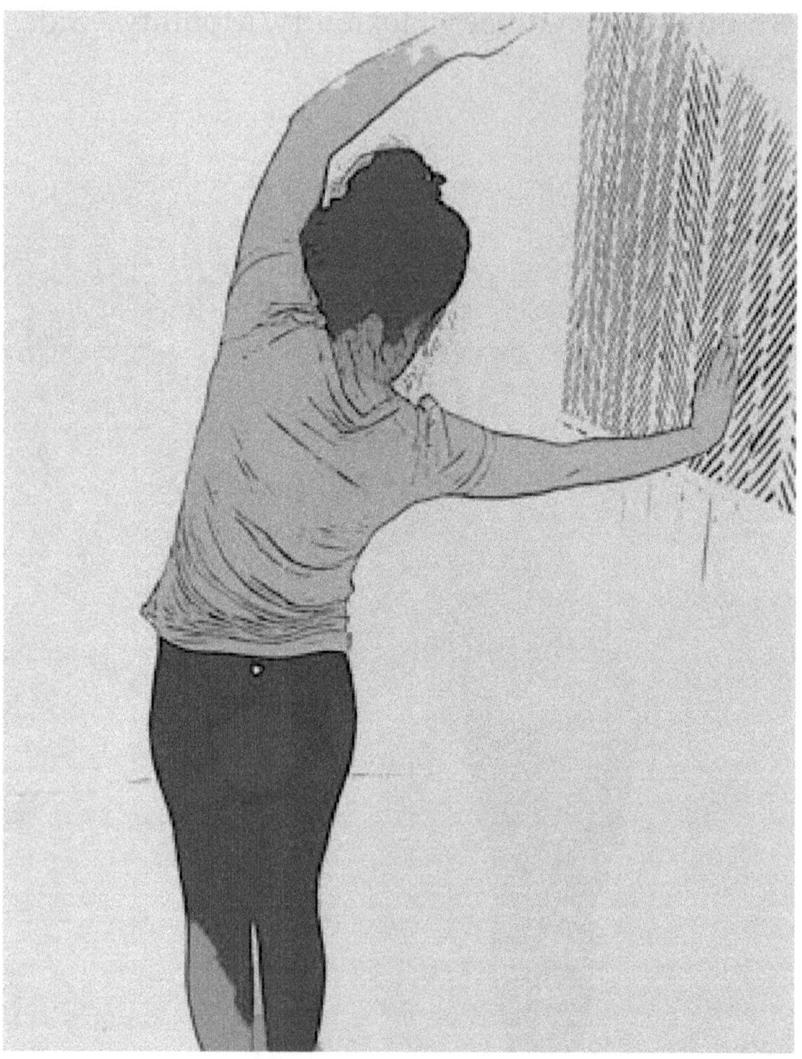

Side Bend - Back View: Stand with right side facing the wall, raise right arm and place hand on wall above head, lean into wall while pushing hips outward, switch sides.

* * *

5th minute: Beginner - Flexibility/Mobility - Reclined Wall Leg Stretch

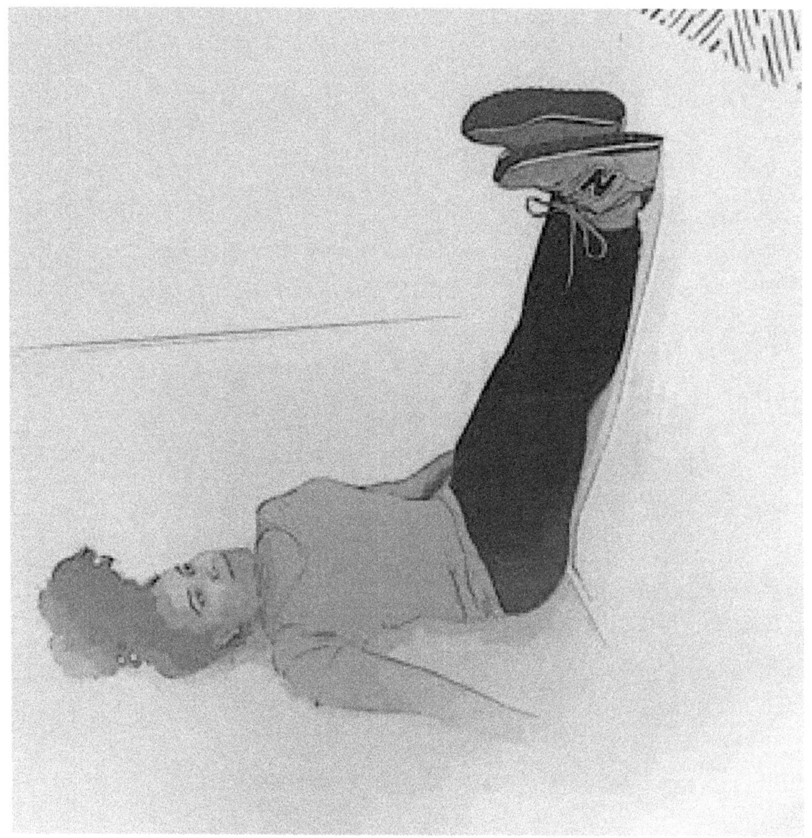

Reclined Wall Leg Stretch: Lie on back with buttocks close to wall, legs extended up, press heels toward ceiling.

III

Intermediate Weekly Plan

This plan is for a 5-minute exercise routine for days Monday through Saturday, tailored to fit a variety of focus areas and intensity levels, ensuring a well-rounded workout experience throughout the week.

Let's turn it up a notch!

Please remember to BREATHE during and between each exercise.

Intermediate Monday

- **1st minute**: Intermediate - Core/Abs - **Wall V-Sit**
- **2nd minute**: Intermediate - Core/Abs - **Wall Leg Raises**
- **3rd minute**: Intermediate - Core/Abs - **Supine Wall Toe Taps**
- **4th minute**: Intermediate - Balance/Stability - **Wall Single-Leg Squat**
- **5th minute**: Intermediate - Balance/Stability - **Wall Warrior III**

See Illustrations and How to Perform Exercise below

* * *

1st minute: Intermediate - Core/Abs - Wall V-Sit

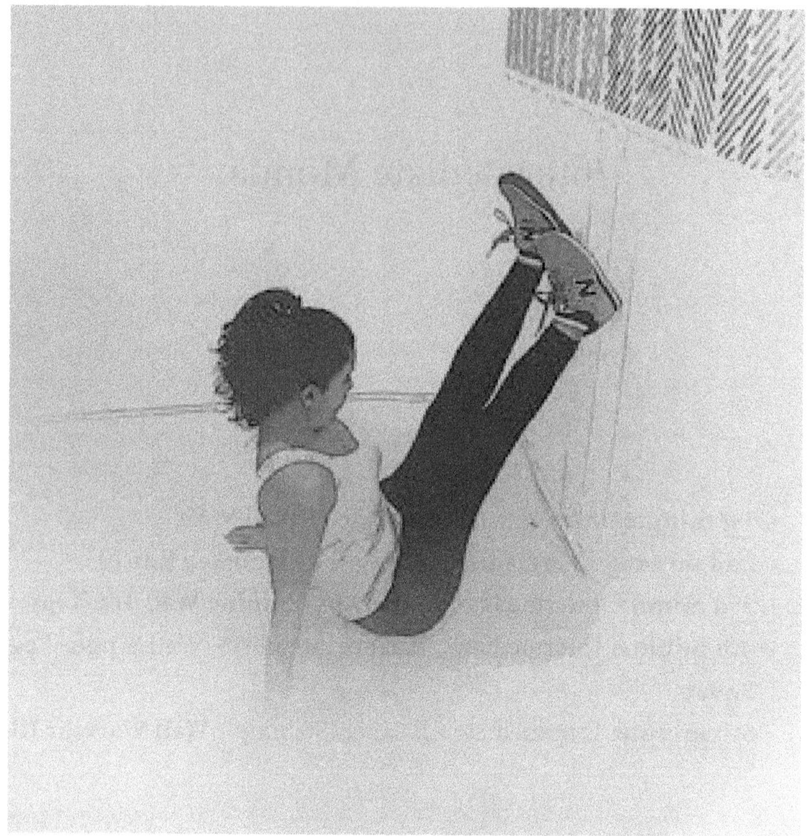

Wall V-Sit: Sit facing wall and place legs going straight up the wall and feet resting at highest point and plant arms behind your back to support the move. Your buttocks should rest between 6-12 inches from base of wall. You should form a tight V shape, hold position.

* * *

2nd minute: Intermediate - Core/Abs - Wall Leg Raises

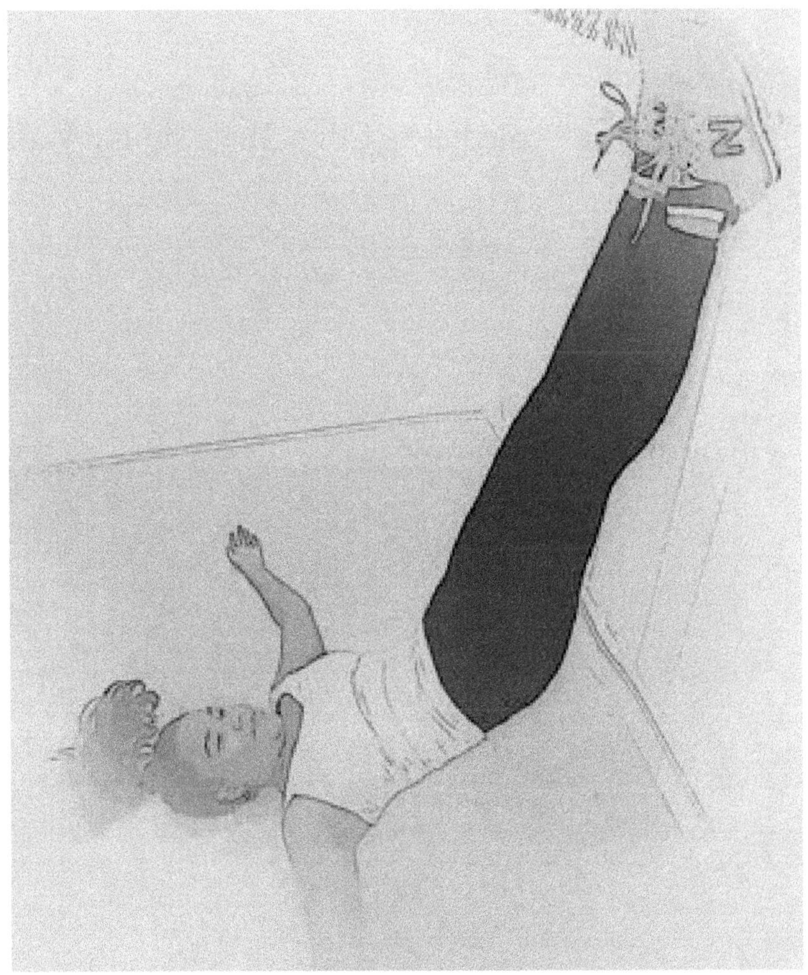

Wall Leg Raises: Lie on back, legs straight up against the wall, lower them towards the ground without touching, lift back up.

* * *

3rd minute: Intermediate - Core/Abs - Supine Wall Toe Taps

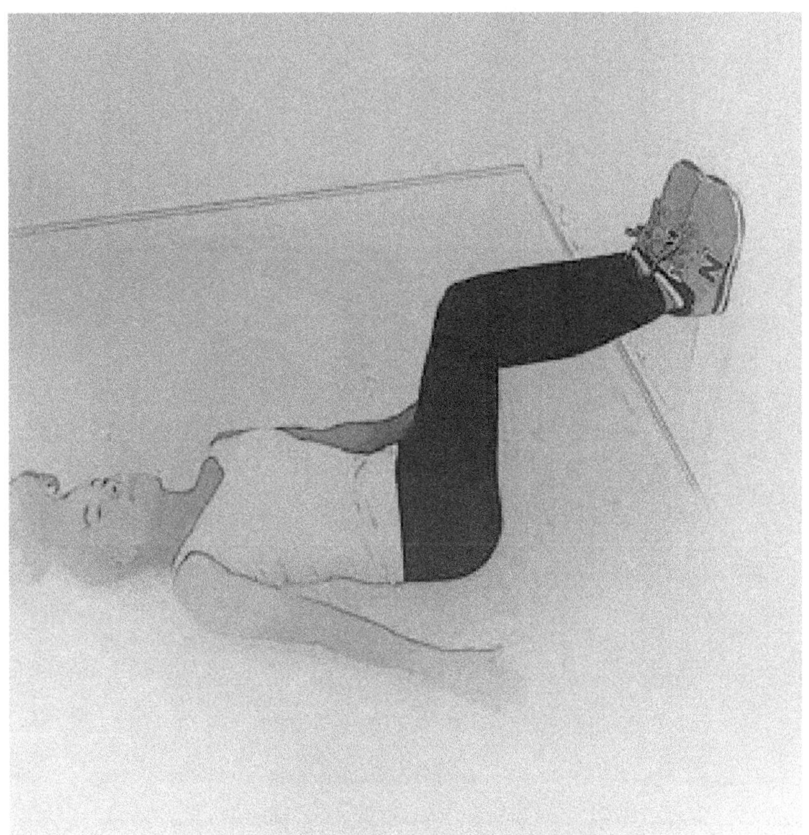

Supine Wall Toe Taps - Part 1: Lie on back, legs raised and pressed against the wall at 90 degree angle

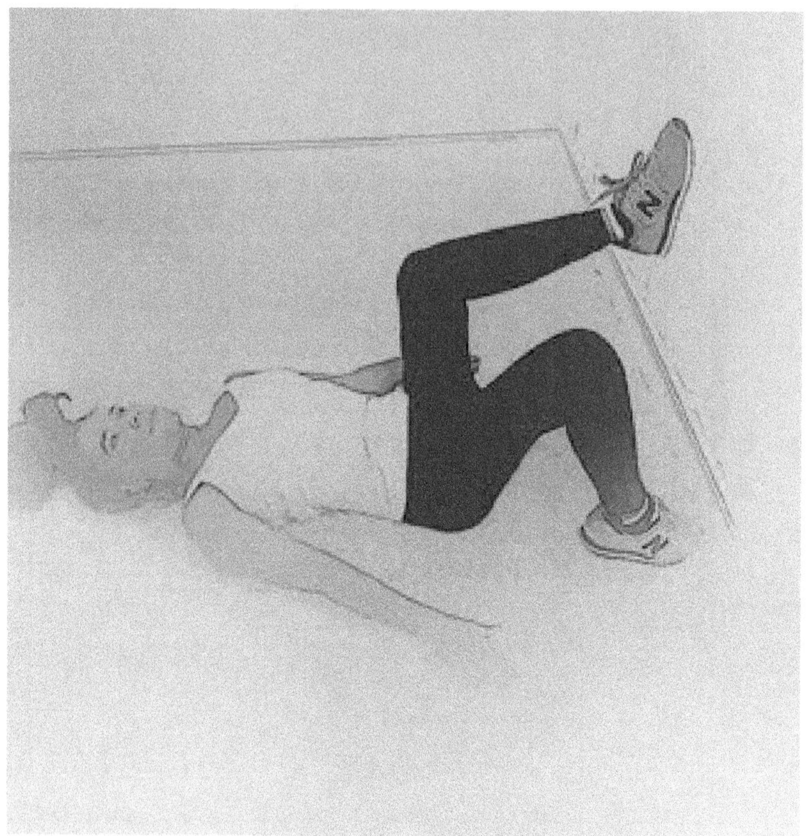

Supine Wall Toe Taps - Part 2: Alternate tapping one foot to the ground at base of wall and lifting the other knee in towards core.

* * *

4th minute: Intermediate - Balance/Stability - Wall Single-Leg Squat

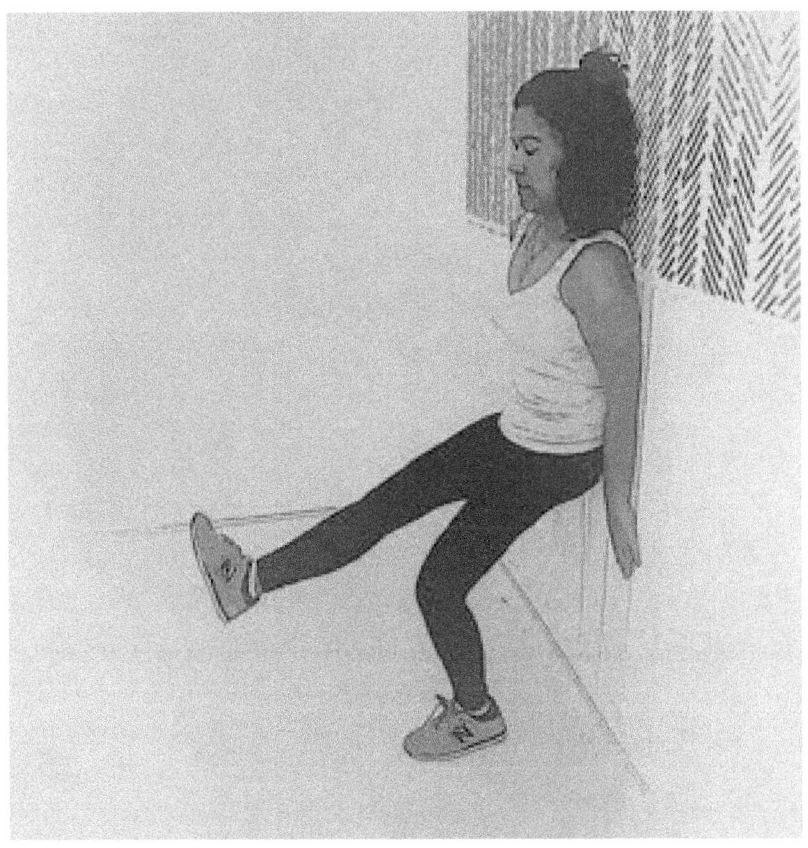

Wall Single-Leg Squat - Part 1: Stand with back to wall for support, slide down to come to squat on one leg, use wall for balance.

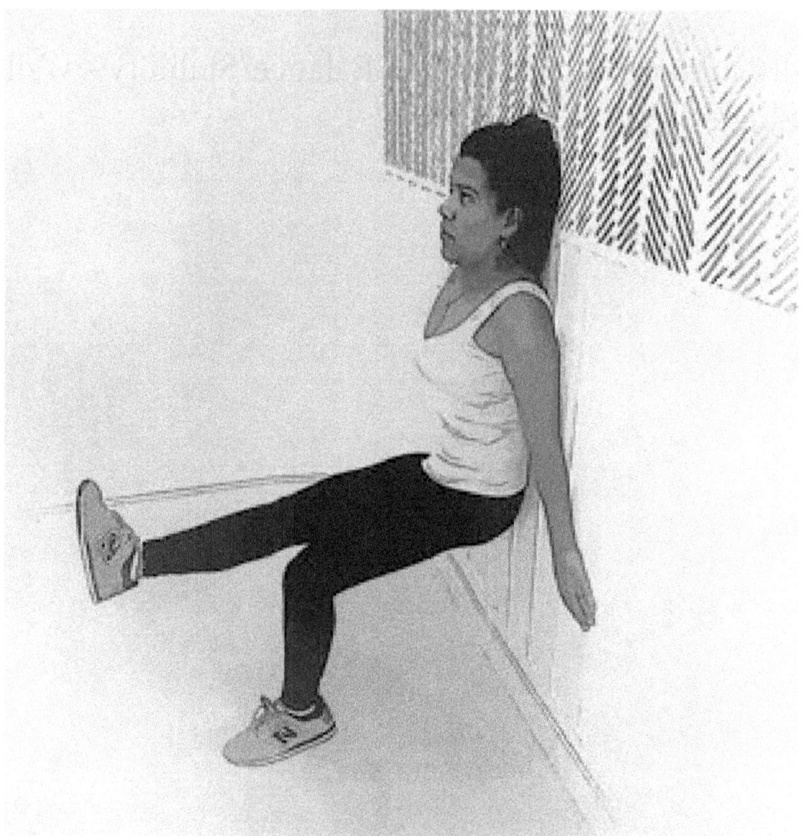

Wall Single-Leg Squat - Part 2: Come into full squat and hold then raise up, switch legs.

* * *

5th minute: Intermediate - Balance/Stability - Wall Warrior III

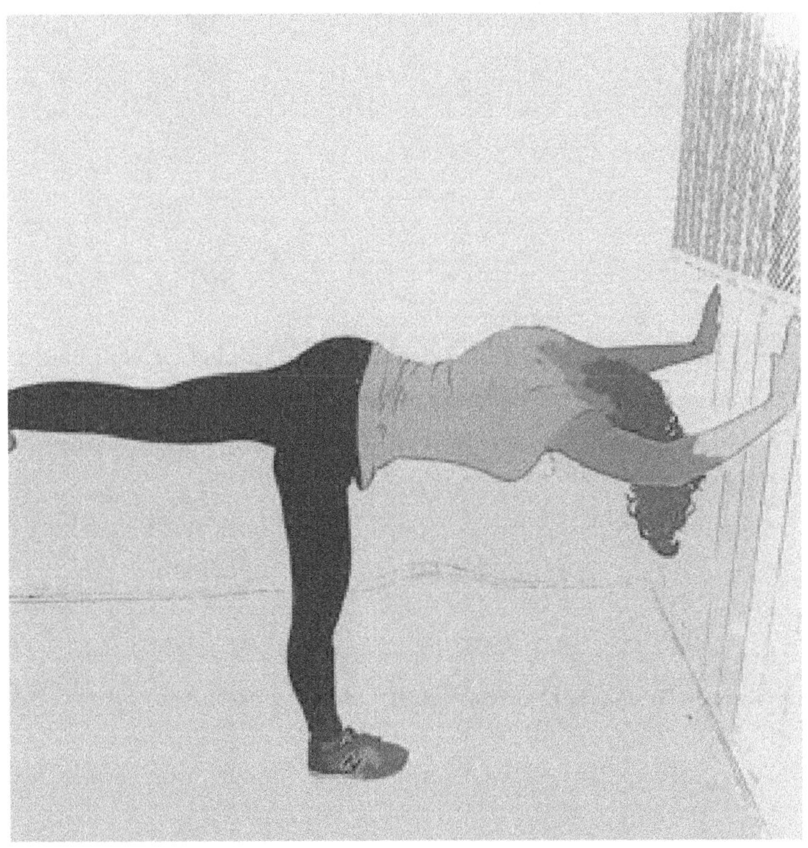

Wall Warrior III Exercise: Stand facing a wall and lean forward, placing your hands on the wall. Stretch one leg back, keeping your body and the extended leg in a straight line. Make sure your leg, back, neck, and arms form a line that's parallel to the floor but at a right angle to the wall. Keep the leg you're standing on straight, aligned with the wall.

Intermediate Tuesday

- **1st minute**: Intermediate - Legs/Glutes - **Single Leg Wall Bridge**
- **2nd minute**: Intermediate - Legs/Glutes - **Wall Lunge**
- **3rd minute**: Intermediate - Legs/Glutes - **Wall Sit With One Leg Extended**
- **4th minute**: Intermediate - Back - **Wall Plank with Arm Lift**
- **5th minute:** Intermediate - Back - **Wall Superman**

See Illustrations and How to Perform Exercise below

* * *

1st minute: Intermediate - Legs/Glutes - Single Leg Wall Bridge

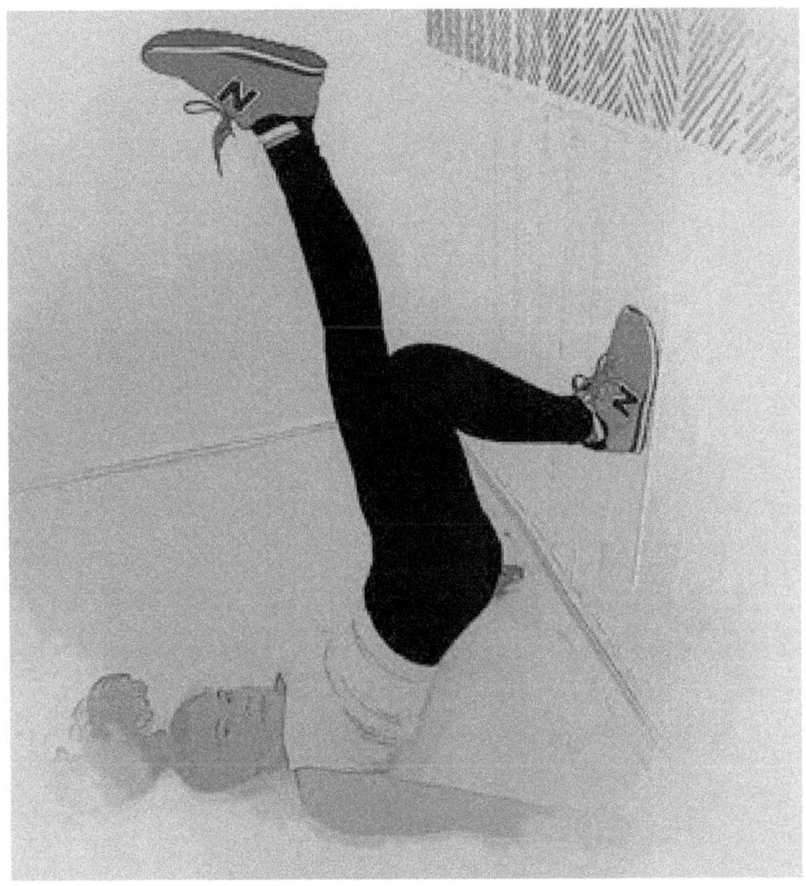

Single Leg Wall Bridge: Lie on back, one foot on wall, other leg extended, lift hips towards ceiling, switch legs.

* * *

2nd minute: Intermediate - Legs/Glutes - Wall Lunge

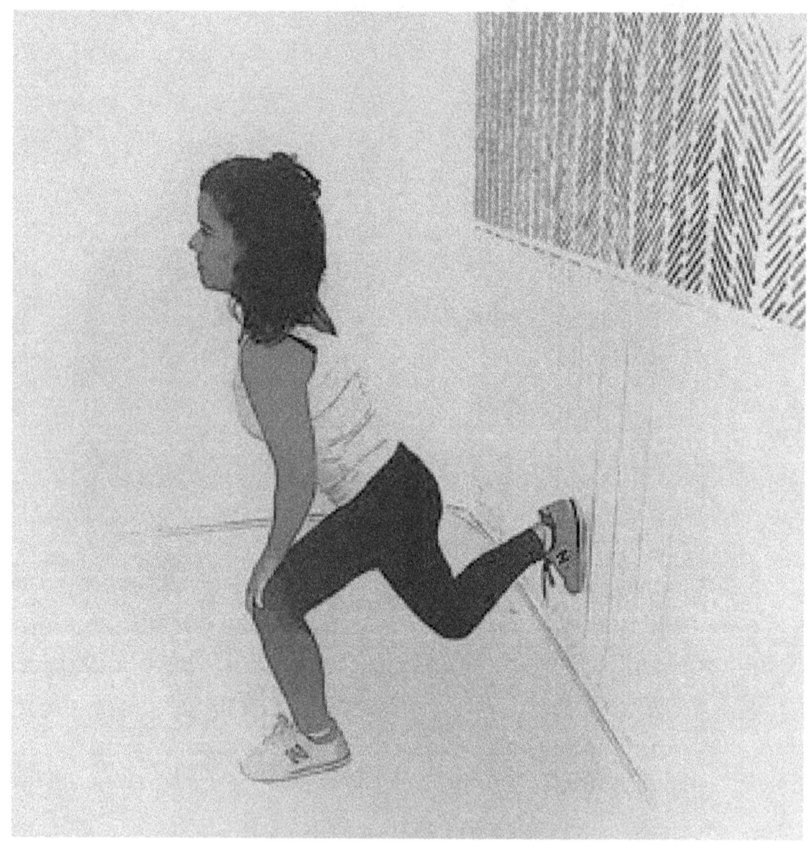

Wall Lunge: Stand with back to wall, one foot placed back against the wall, lunge forward with the other leg, return to start, switch legs.

* * *

3rd minute: Intermediate - Legs/Glutes - Wall Sit With One Leg Extended

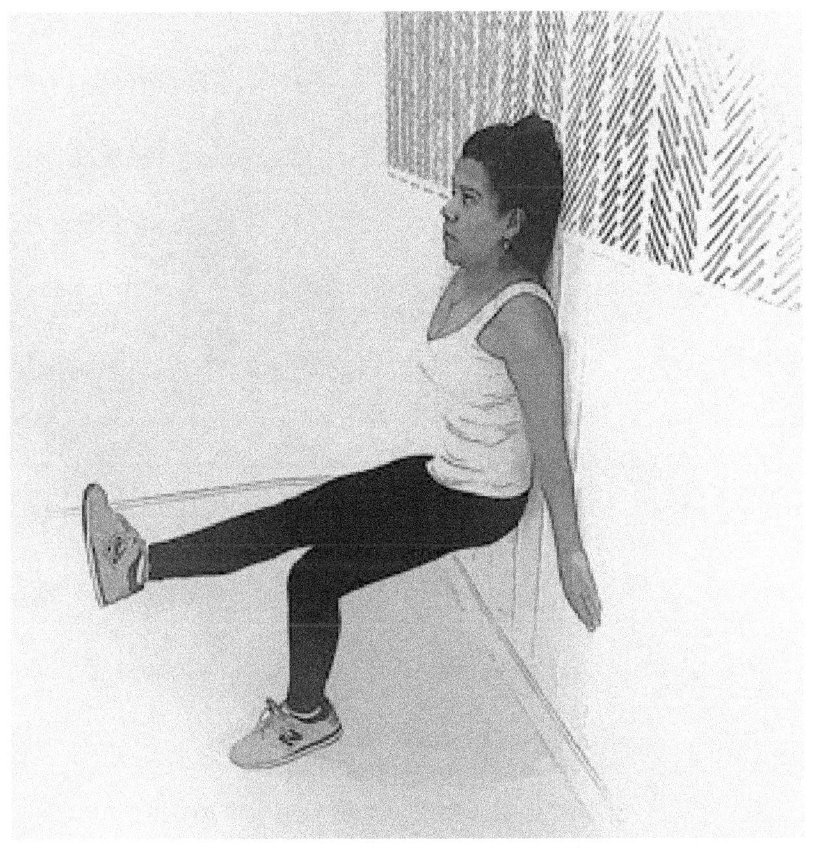

* * *

4th minute: Intermediate - Back - Wall Plank with Arm Lift

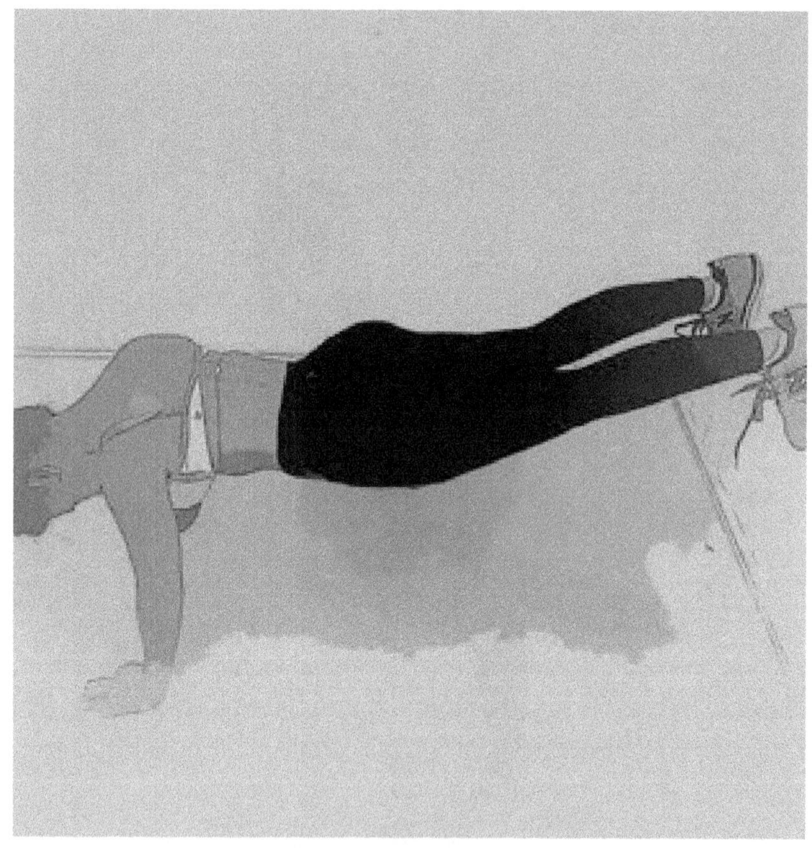

Wall Plank with Arm Lift: In a plank position with feet on the wall, alternate lifting each arm, keeping core engaged.

* * *

5th minute: Intermediate - Back - Wall Superman

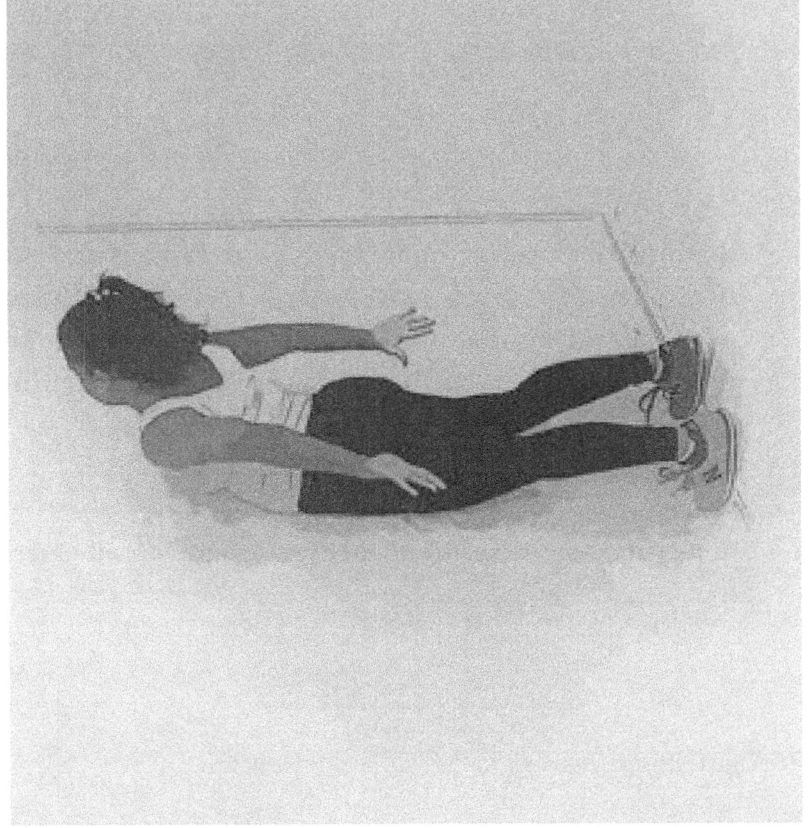

Wall Superman: Lie face down, feet against the wall, lift arms and legs off the ground, hold, lower back down.

Intermediate Wednesday

- **1st minute**: Intermediate - Upper Body - **Wall Plank with Arm Lift**
- **2nd minute**: Intermediate - Upper Body - **Wall Superman**
- **3rd minute**: Intermediate - Upper Body - **Wall Forearm Push-Up**
- **4th minute**: Intermediate - Flexibility/Mobility - **Wall Pike Stretch**
- **5th minute**: Intermediate - Flexibility/Mobility - **Wall Quad Stretch**

See Illustrations and How to Perform Exercise below

* * *

1st minute: Intermediate - Upper Body - Wall Plank with Arm Lift

75

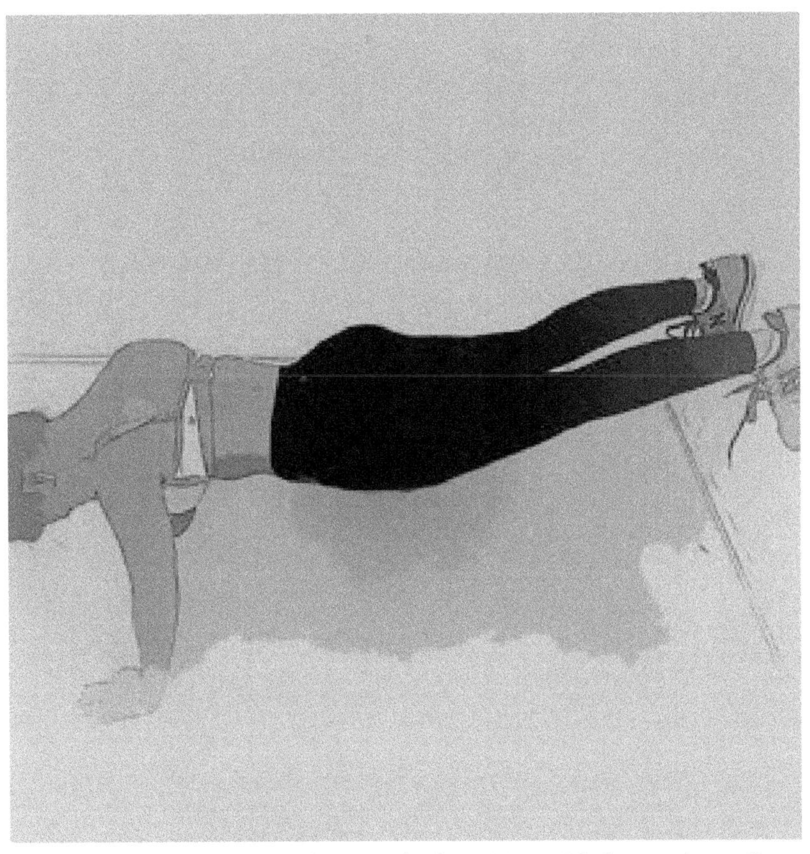

Wall Plank with Arm Lift: In a plank position with feet on the wall, alternate lifting each arm, keeping core engaged.

* * *

2nd minute: Intermediate - Upper Body - Wall Superman

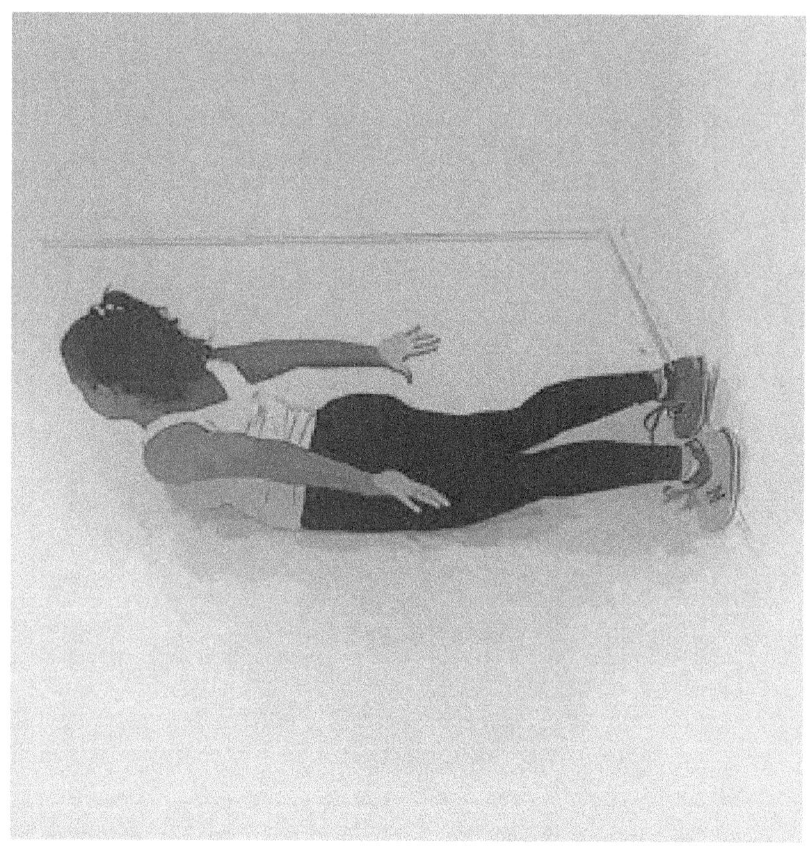

Wall Superman: Lie face down, feet against the lower wall, lift arms and legs off the ground, hold, lower back down, face pointing semi-downward.

* * *

3rd minute: Intermediate - Upper Body - Wall Forearm Push-Up

77

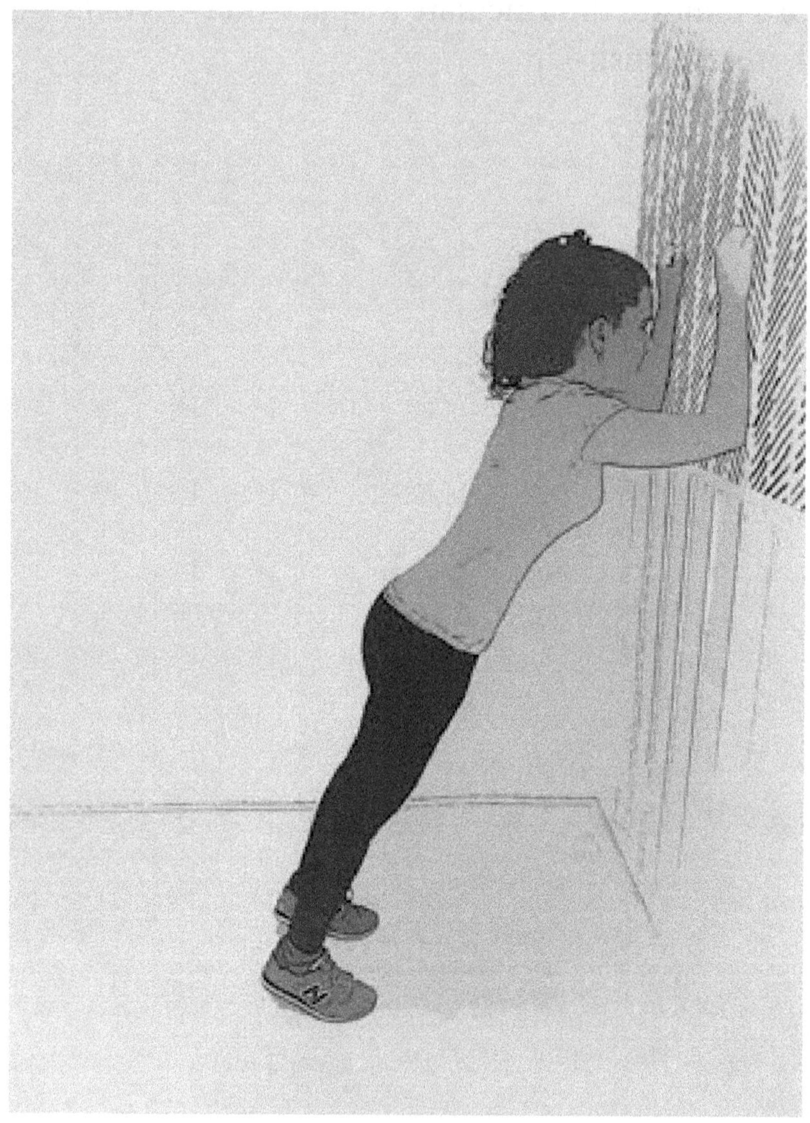

Wall Forearm Push-Up - Part 1: Face the wall, place forearms on the wall.

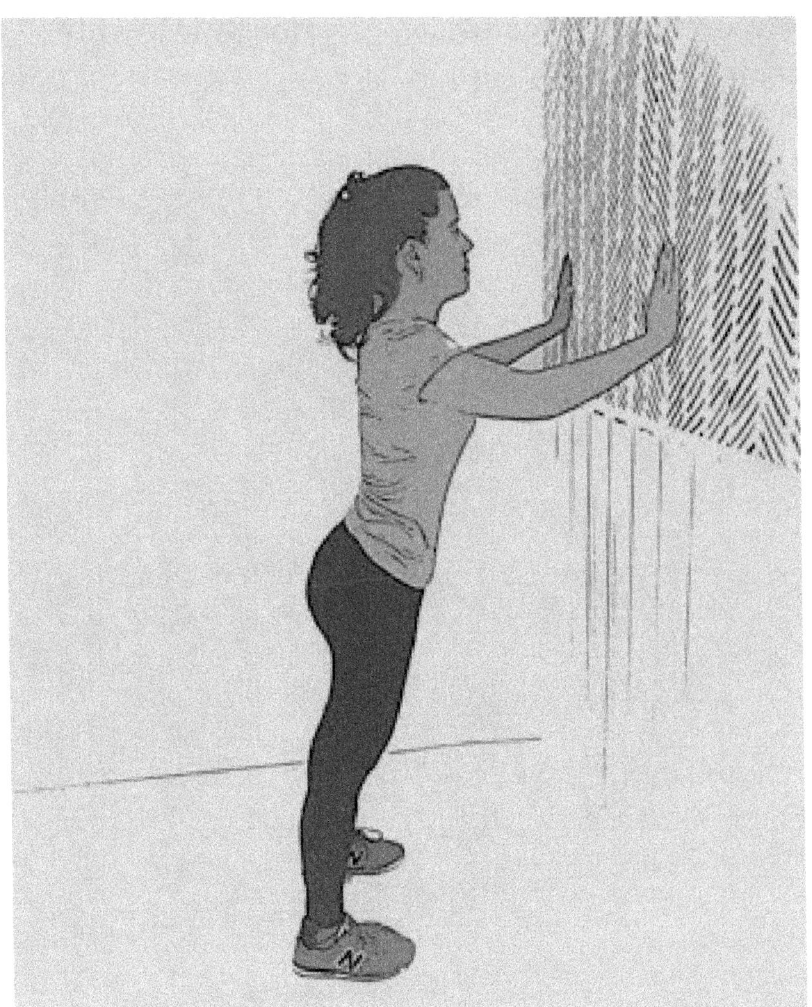

Wall Forearm Push-Up - Part 2: Push off with your arms to engage upper body.

* * *

4th minute: Intermediate - Flexibility/Mobility - Wall Pike Stretch

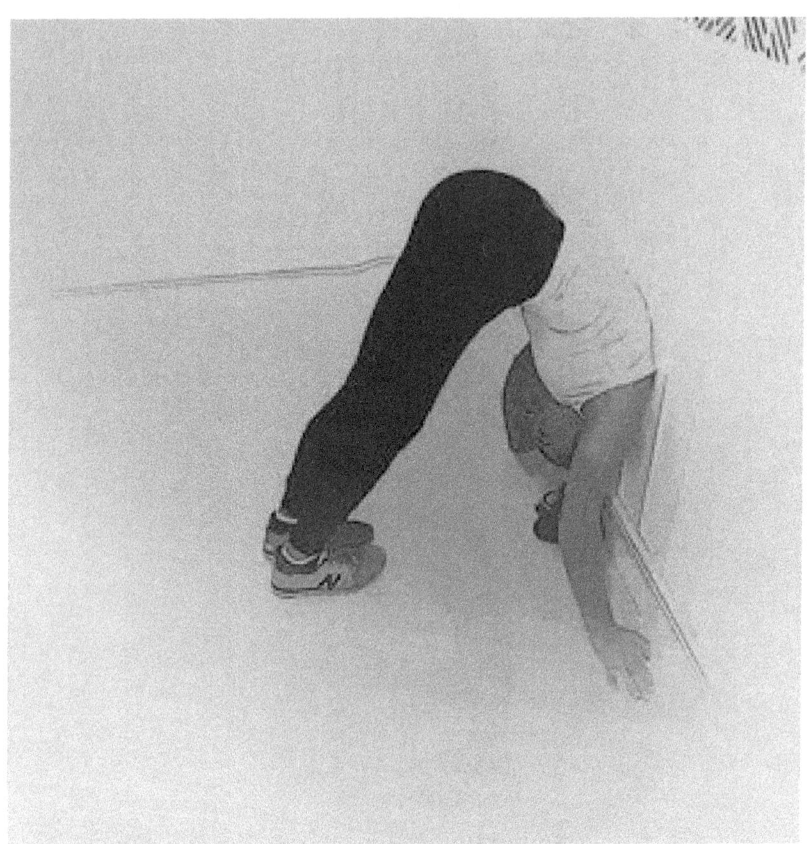

Wall Pike Stretch: Stand facing wall, bend over and reach hands towards ground, hold stretch with wall supporting extension while piking hips.

* * *

5th minute: Intermediate - Flexibility/Mobility - Wall Quad Stretch

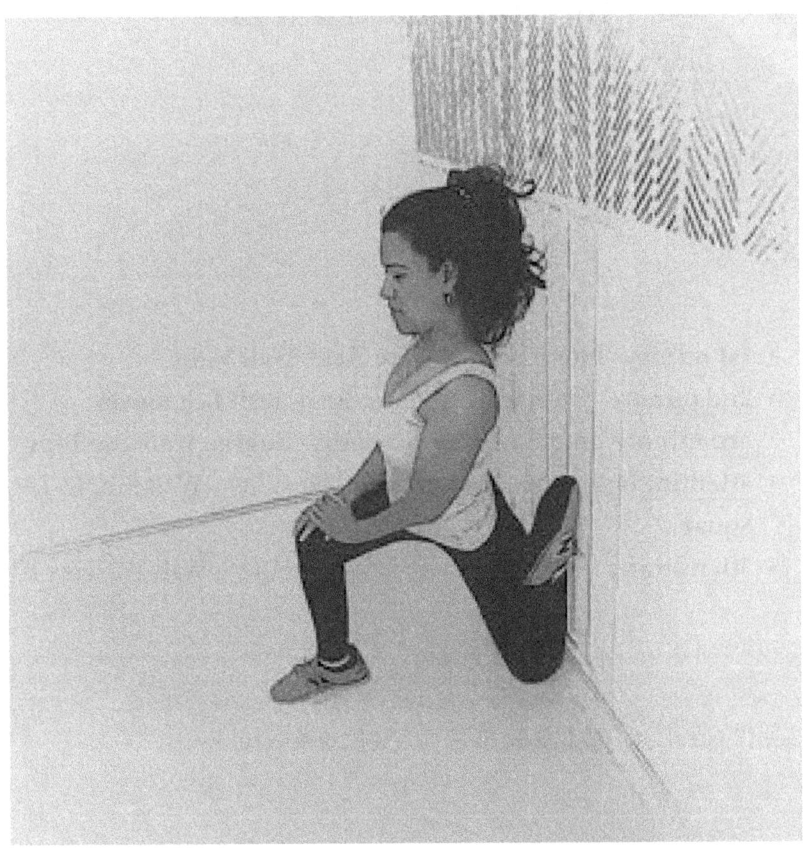

Wall Quad Stretch: Stand facing away from wall, place one foot on wall behind you, push hips forward, hold, switch legs.

Intermediate Thursday

- **1st minute**: Intermediate - Core/Abs - **Wall V-Sit**
- **2nd minute**: Intermediate - Core/Abs - **Wall Leg Raises**
- **3rd minute**: Intermediate - Core/Abs - **Supine Wall Toe Taps**
- **4th minute**: Intermediate - Balance/Stability - **Wall Single-Leg Squat**
- **5th minute**: Intermediate - Balance/Stability - **Wall Warrior III**

See Illustrations and How to Perform Exercise below

* * *

1st minute: Intermediate - Core/Abs - Wall V-Sit

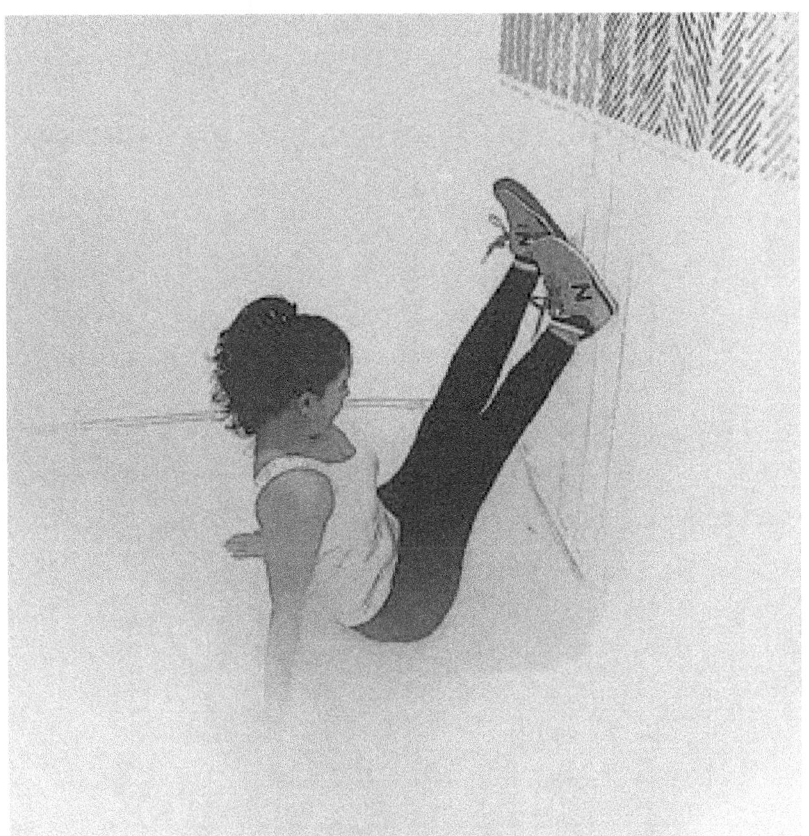

Wall V-Sit: Sit facing wall and place legs going straight up the wall and feet resting at highest point and plant arms behind your back to support the move. Your buttocks should rest between 6-12 inches from base of wall. You should form a tight V shape, hold position.

* * *

2nd minute: Intermediate - Core/Abs - Wall Leg Raises

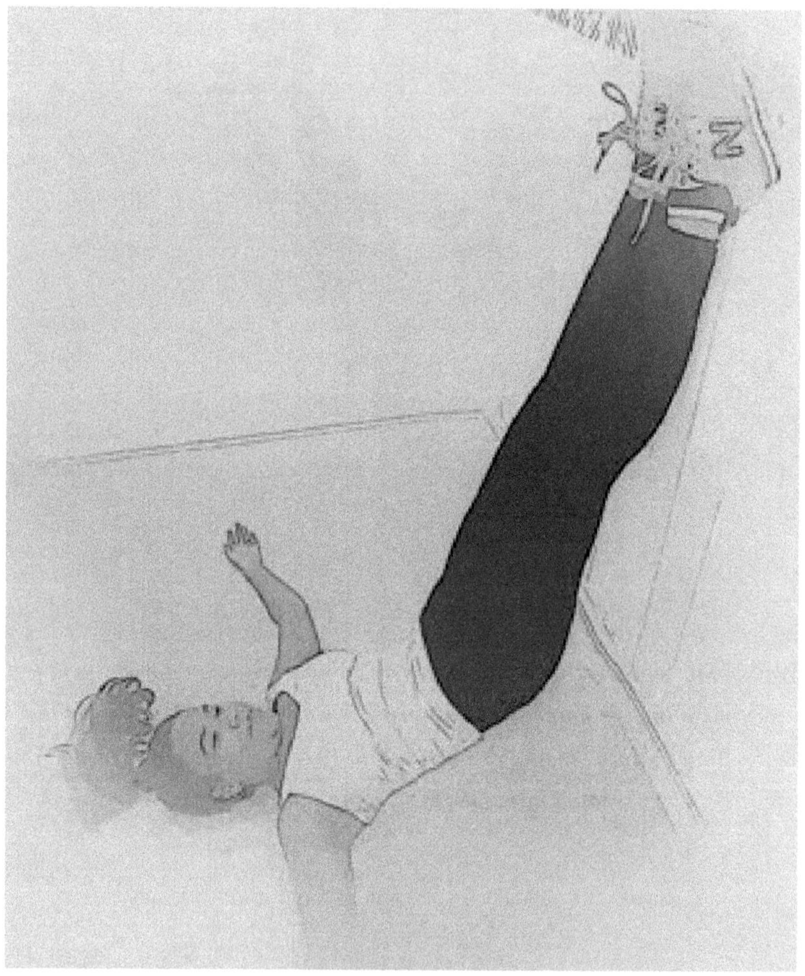

Wall Leg Raises: Lie on back, legs straight up against the wall, lower them towards the ground without touching, lift back up.

* * *

3rd minute: Intermediate - Core/Abs - Supine Wall Toe Taps

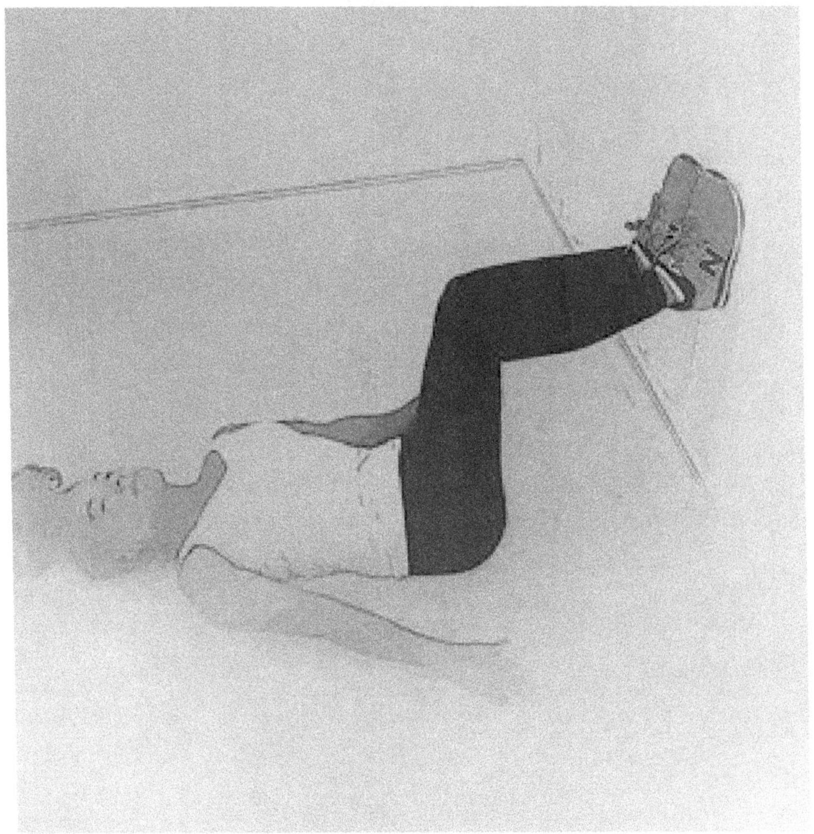

Supine Wall Toe Taps - Part 1: Lie on back, legs raised and pressed against the wall at 90 degree angle

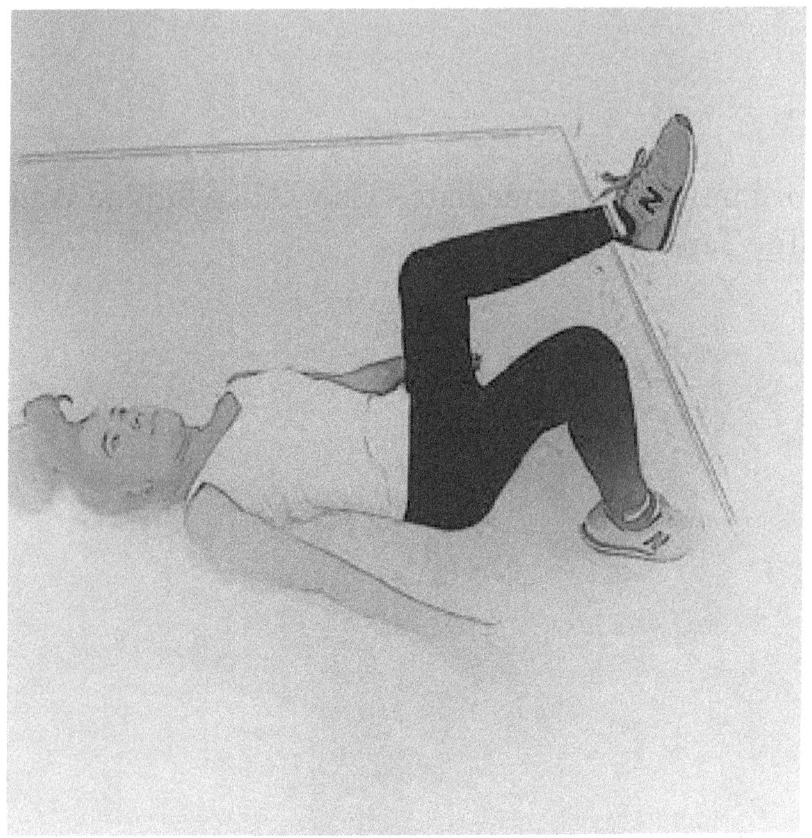

Supine Wall Toe Taps - Part 2: Alternate tapping one foot to the ground at base of wall and lifting the other knee in towards core.

* * *

4th minute: Intermediate - Balance/Stability - Wall Single-Leg Squat

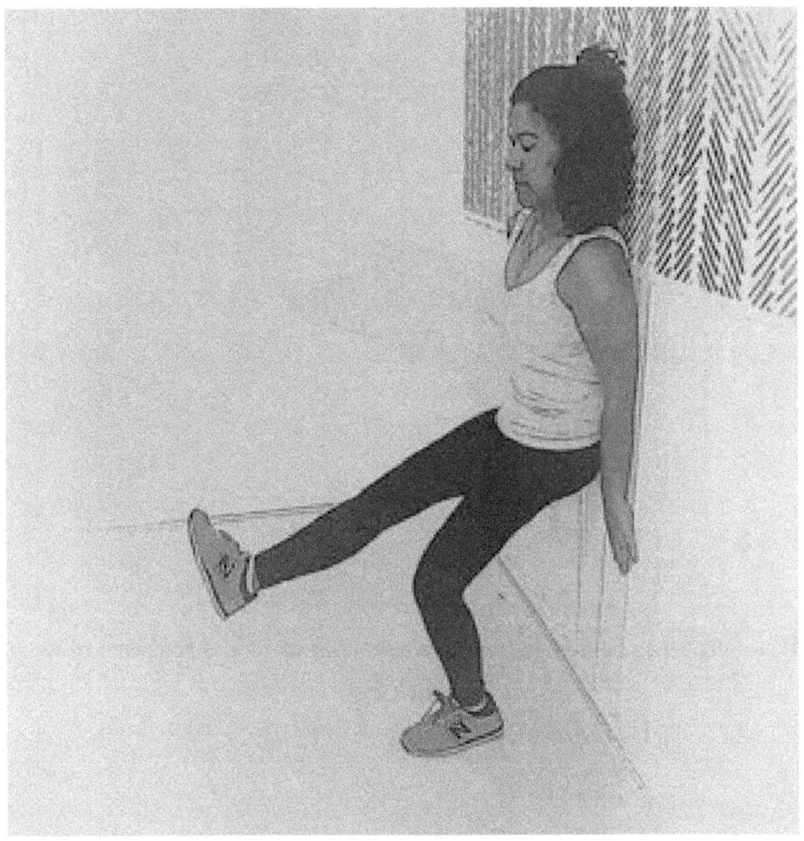

Wall Single-Leg Squat - Part 1: Stand with back to wall for support, slide down to come to squat on one leg, use wall for balance.

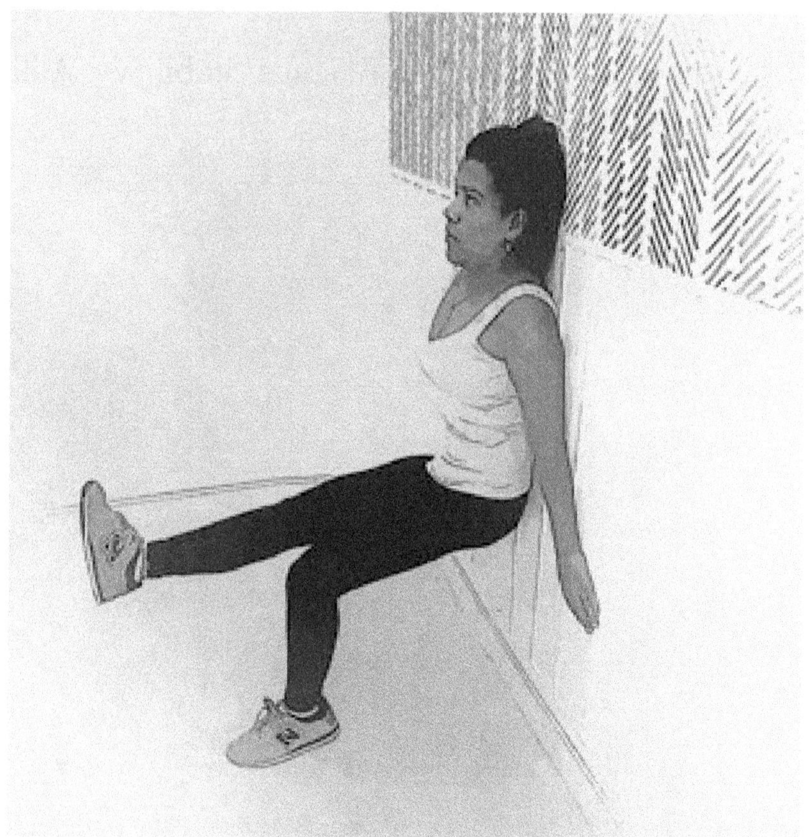

Wall Single-Leg Squat - Part 2: Come into full squat and hold then raise up, switch legs.

* * *

5th minute: Intermediate - Balance/Stability - Wall Warrior III

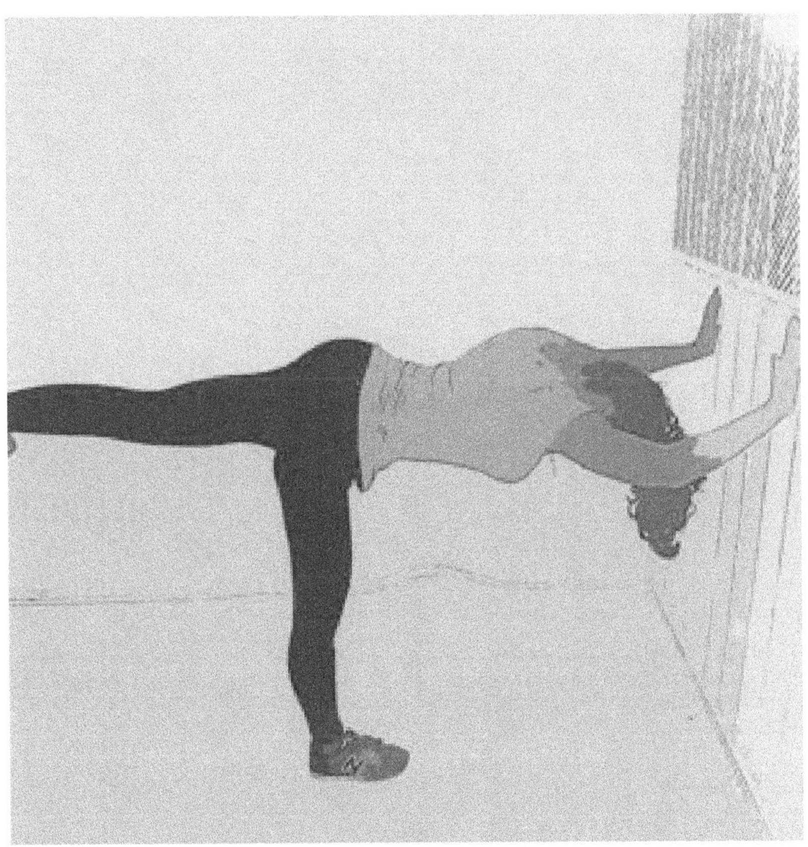

Wall Warrior III Exercise: Stand facing a wall and lean forward, placing your hands on the wall. Stretch one leg back, keeping your body and the extended leg in a straight line. Make sure your leg, back, neck, and arms form a line that's parallel to the floor but at a right angle to the wall. Keep the leg you're standing on straight, aligned with the wall.

Intermediate Friday

- **1st minute**: Intermediate - Legs/Glutes - **Single Leg Wall Bridge**
- **2nd minute**: Intermediate - Legs/Glutes - **Wall Lunge**
- **3rd minute**: Intermediate - Legs/Glutes - **Wall Sit With One Leg Extended**
- **4th minute**: Intermediate - Back - **Wall Plank with Arm Lift**
- **5th minute**: Intermediate - Back - **Wall Superman**

See Illustrations and How to Perform Exercise below

* * *

1st minute: Intermediate - Legs/Glutes - Single Leg Wall Bridge

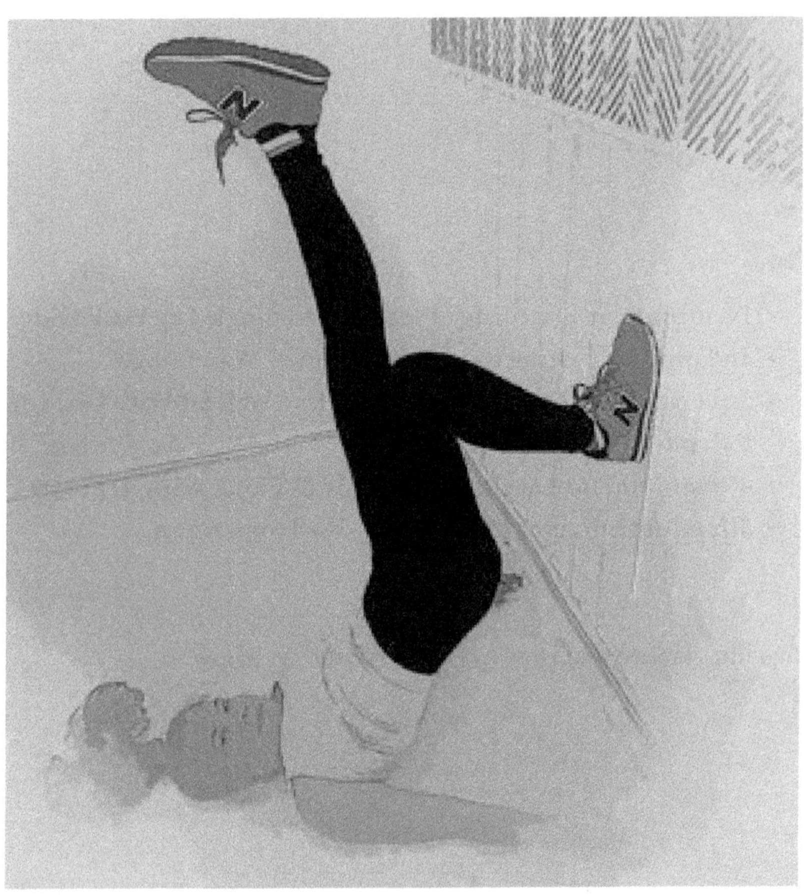

Single Leg Wall Bridge: Lie on back, one foot on wall, other leg extended, lift hips towards ceiling, switch legs.

* * *

2nd minute: Intermediate - Legs/Glutes - Wall Lunge

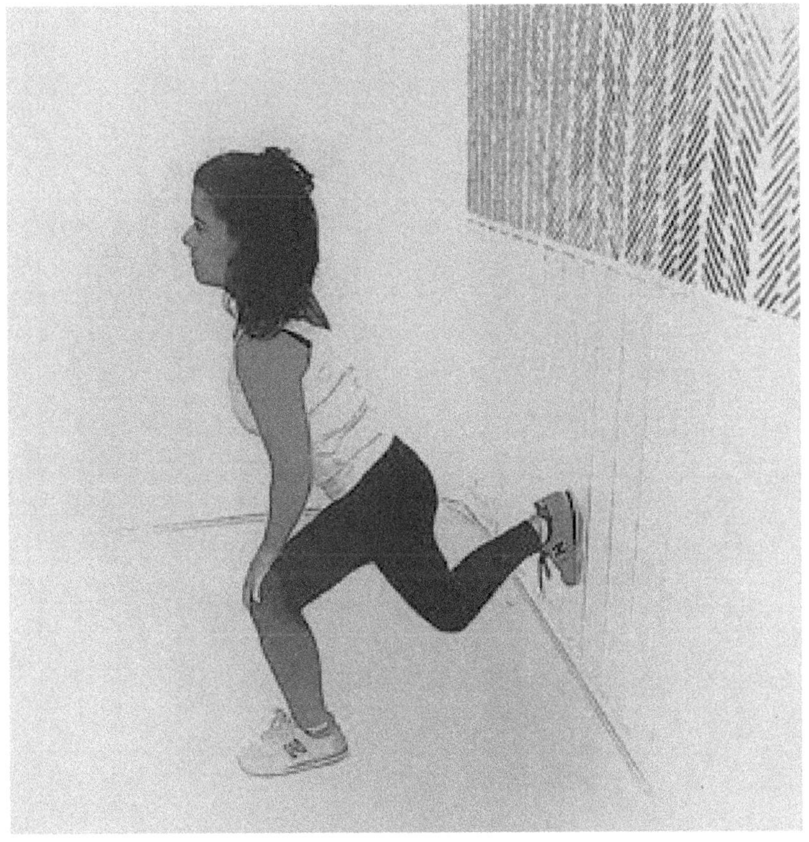

Wall Lunge: Stand with back to wall, one foot placed back against the wall, lunge forward with the other leg, return to start, switch legs.

* * *

3rd minute: Intermediate - Legs/Glutes - Wall Sit With One Leg Extended

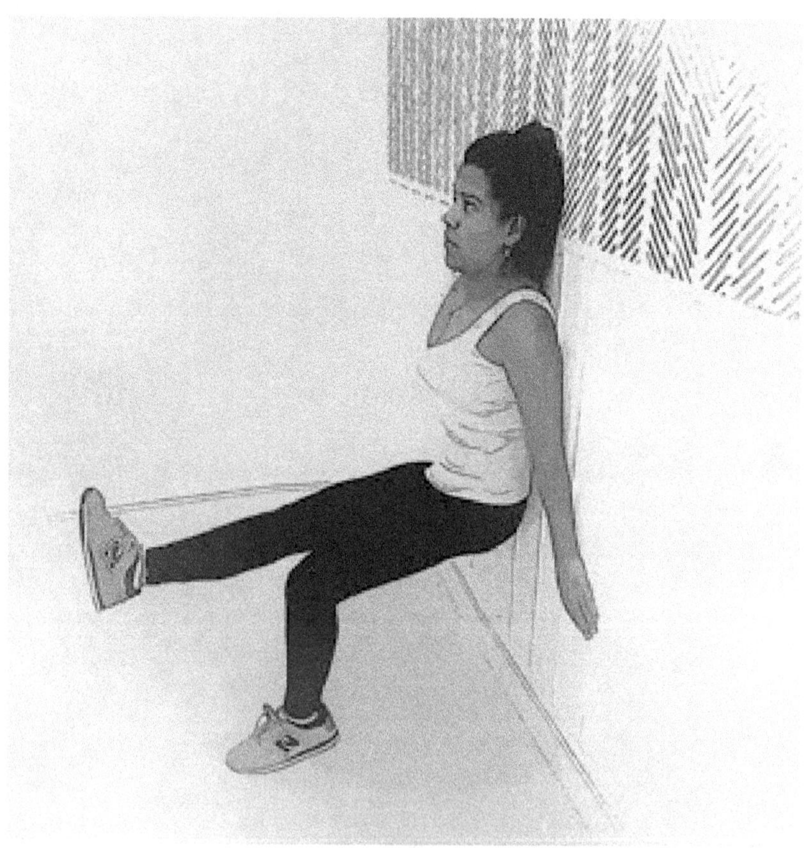

* * *

4th minute: Intermediate - Back - Wall Plank with Arm Lift

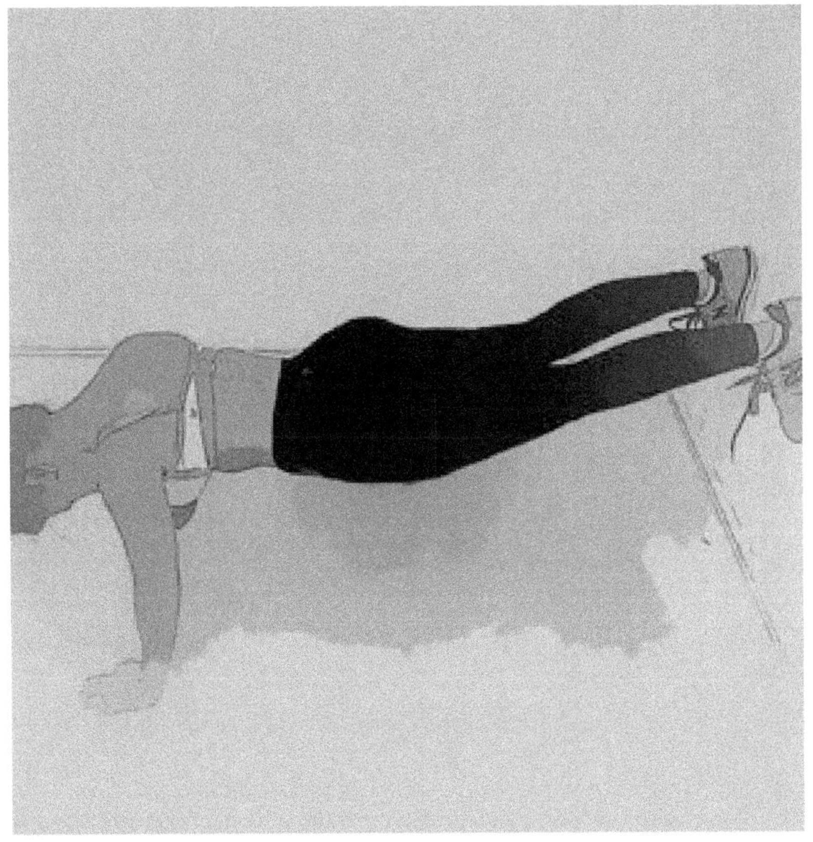

Wall Plank with Arm Lift: In a plank position with feet on the wall, alternate lifting each arm, keeping core engaged.

* * *

5th minute: Intermediate - Back - Wall Superman

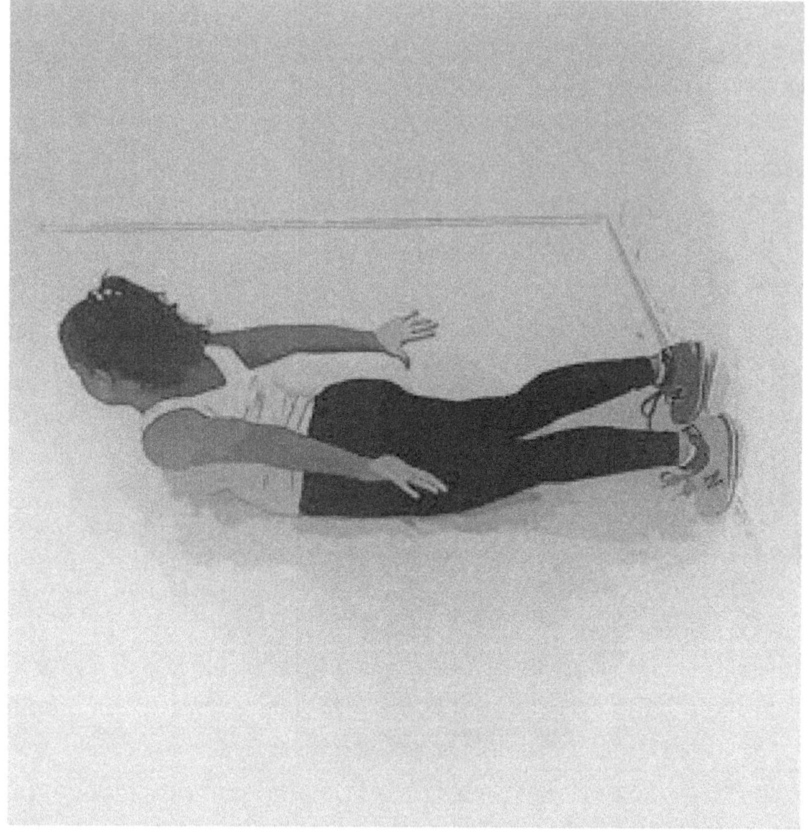

Wall Superman: Lie face down, feet against the wall, lift arms and legs off the ground, hold, lower back down.

INTERMEDIATE FRIDAY

Intermediate Saturday

- **1st minute**: Intermediate - Upper Body - **Wall Plank with Arm Lift**
- **2nd minute**: Intermediate - Upper Body - **Wall Superman**
- **3rd minute**: Intermediate - Upper Body - **Wall Forearm Push-Up**
- **4th minute**: Intermediate - Flexibility/Mobility - **Wall Pike Stretch**
- **5th minute**: Intermediate - Flexibility/Mobility - **Wall Quad Stretch**

See Illustrations and How to Perform Exercise below

* * *

1st minute: Intermediate - Upper Body - Wall Plank with Arm Lift

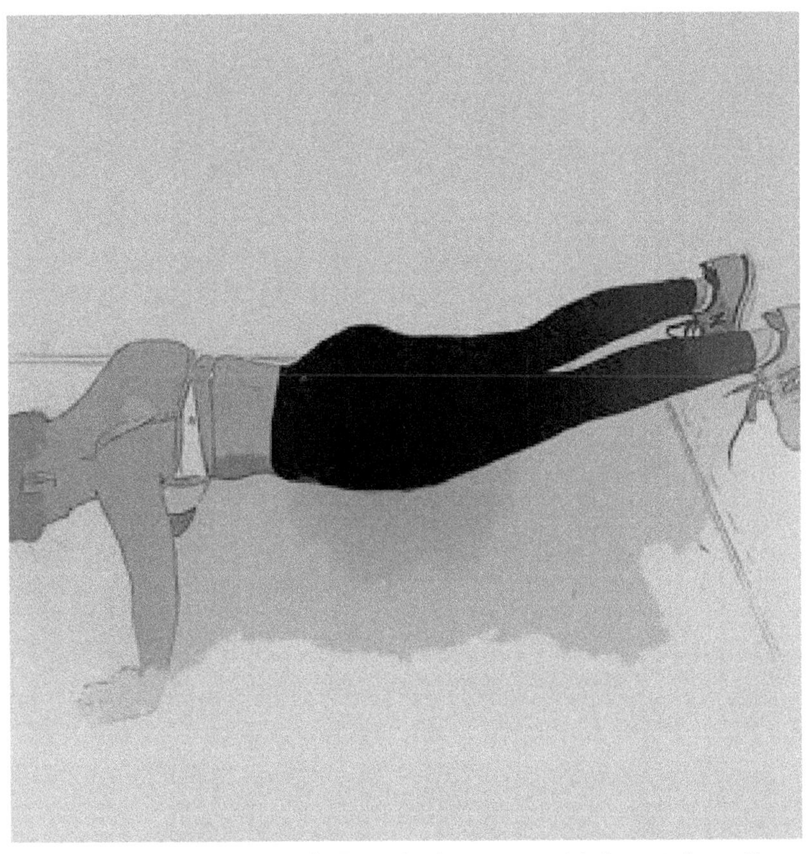

Wall Plank with Arm Lift: In a plank position with feet on the wall, alternate lifting each arm, keeping core engaged.

* * *

2nd minute: Intermediate - Upper Body - Wall Superman

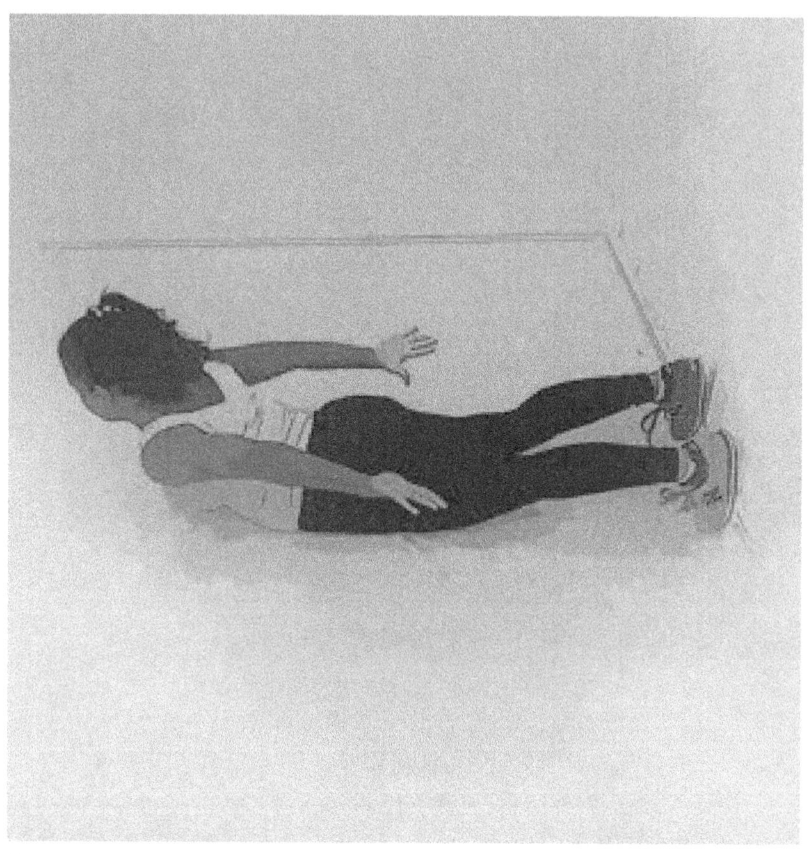

Wall Superman: Lie face down, feet against the lower wall, lift arms and legs off the ground, hold, lower back down, face pointing semi-downward.

* * *

3rd minute: Intermediate - Upper Body - Wall Forearm Push-Up

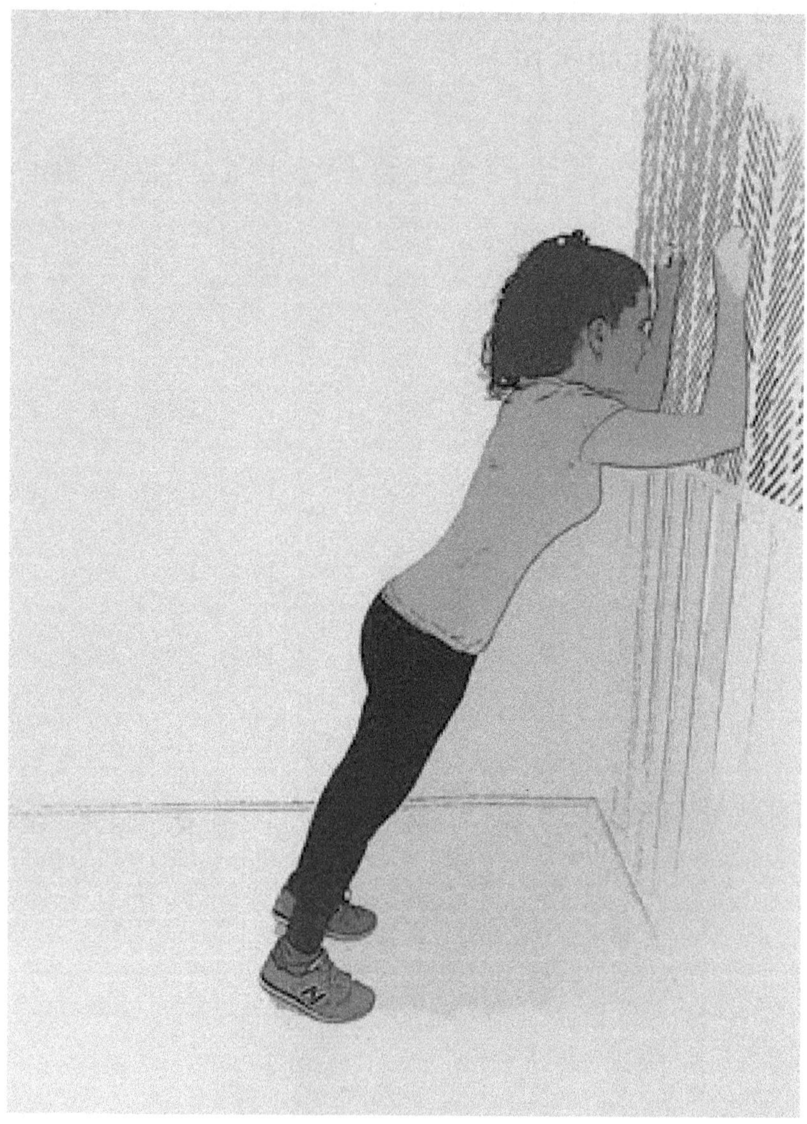

Wall Forearm Push-Up - Part 1: Face the wall, place forearms on the wall.

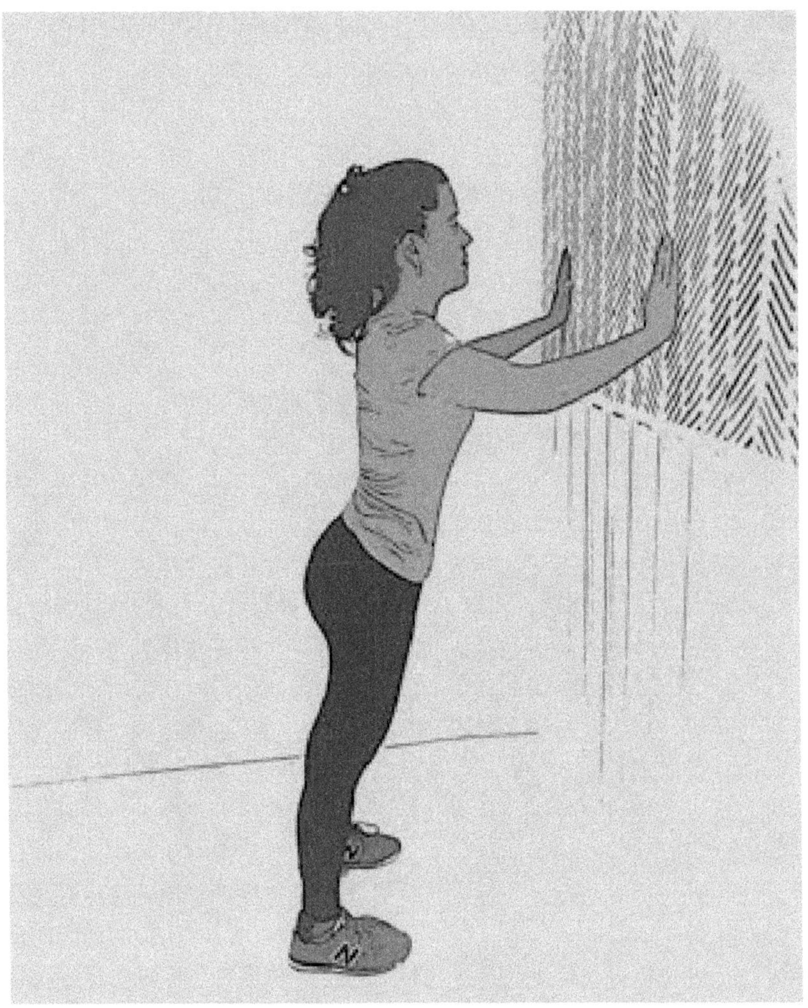

Wall Forearm Push-Up - Part 2: Push off with your arms to engage upper body.

* * *

4th minute: Intermediate - Flexibility/Mobility - Wall Pike Stretch

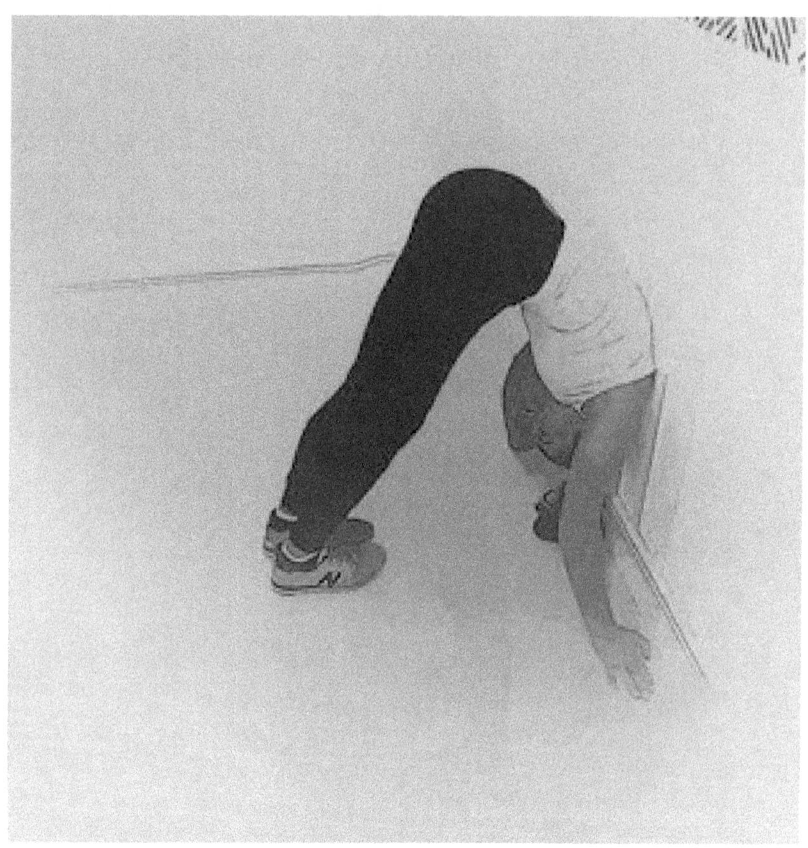

Wall Pike Stretch: Stand facing wall, bend over and reach hands towards ground, hold stretch with wall supporting extension while piking hips.

* * *

5th minute: Intermediate - Flexibility/Mobility - Wall Quad Stretch

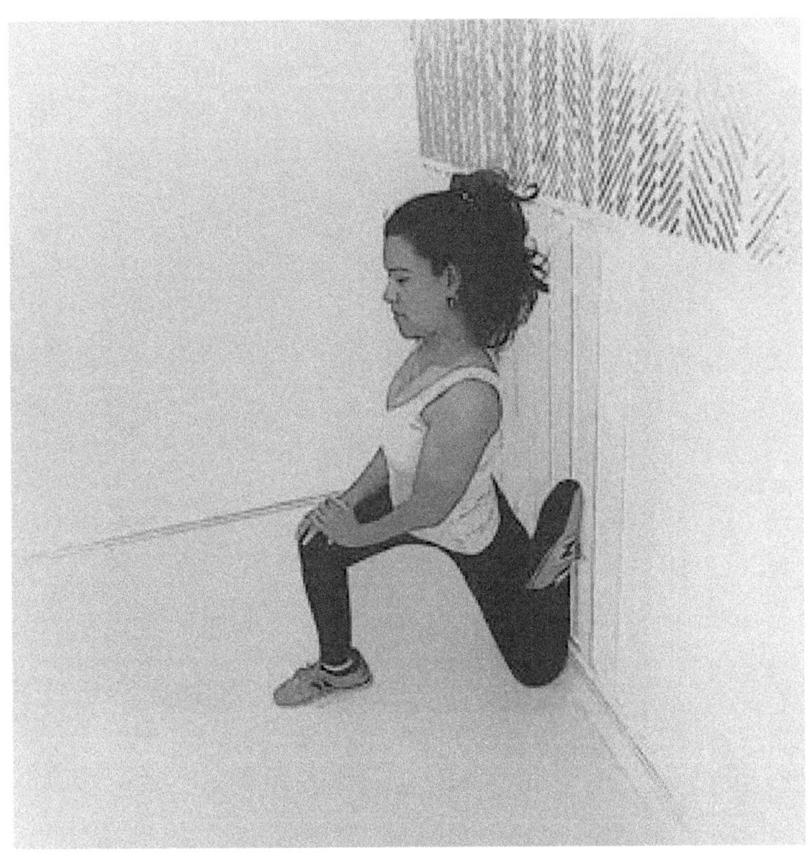

Wall Quad Stretch: Stand facing away from wall, place one foot on wall behind you, push hips forward, hold, switch legs.

IV

Advanced Weekly Plan

This plan is for a 5-minute exercise routine for days Monday through Saturday, tailored to fit a variety of focus areas and intensity levels, ensuring a well-rounded workout experience throughout the week.

Go all out and embrace Wall Pilates in all its wonder!

Please remember to BREATHE during and between each exercise.

Advanced Monday

- **1st minute:** Advanced - Core/Abs - **Inverted Wall Mountain Climbers**
- **2nd minute:** Advanced - Core/Abs - **Wall Scissor Kicks**
- **3rd minute:** Advanced - Core/Abs - **Wall Abdominal Curl**
- **4th minute:** Advanced - Balance/Stability - **Wall Handstand**
- **5th minute:** Advanced - Balance/Stability - **Wall One-Arm Handstand**

See Illustrations and How to Perform Exercise below

* * *

1st minute: Advanced - Core/Abs - Inverted Wall Mountain Climbers

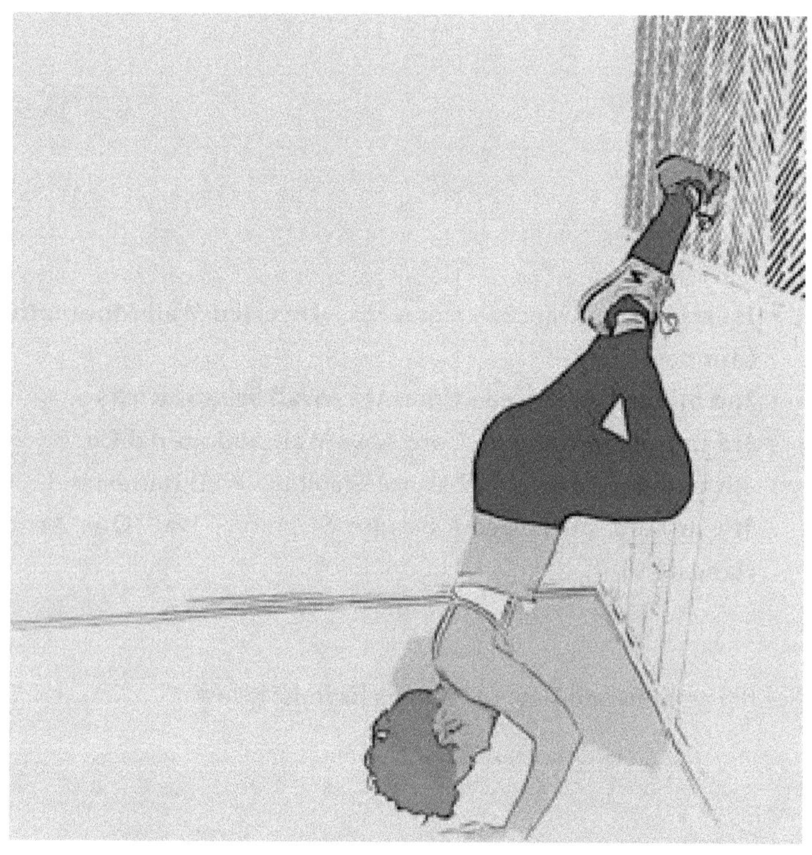

Inverted Wall Mountain Climbers: In a handstand against the wall, alternate driving knees towards chest in a controlled manner.

* * *

2nd minute: Advanced - Core/Abs - Wall Scissor Kicks

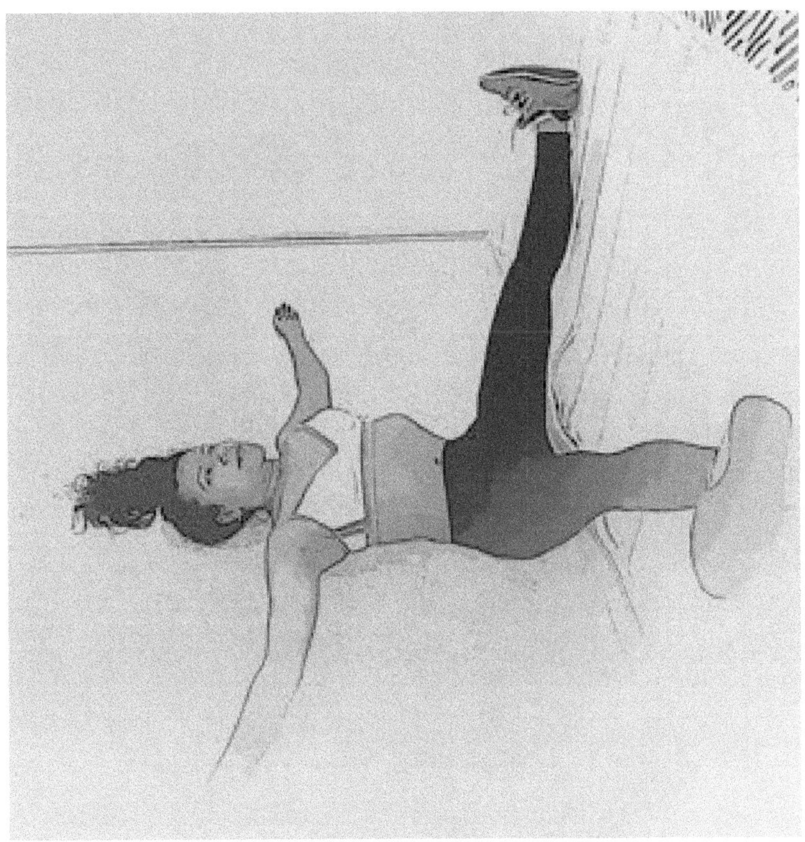

Wall Scissor Kicks: Lie on back, legs up against the wall, perform scissor kicks by alternating leg positions.

* * *

3rd minute: Advanced - Core/Abs - Wall Abdominal Curl

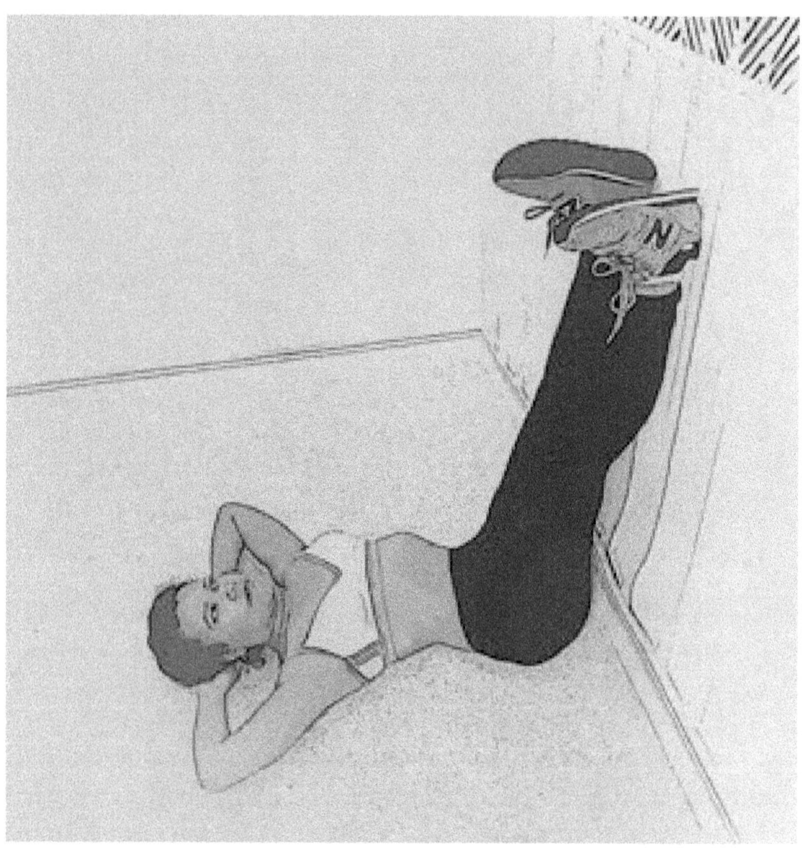

Abdominal Curl - Part 1: Lay down with back against the floor, buttocks on the wall with legs extending vertically along wall toward ceiling.

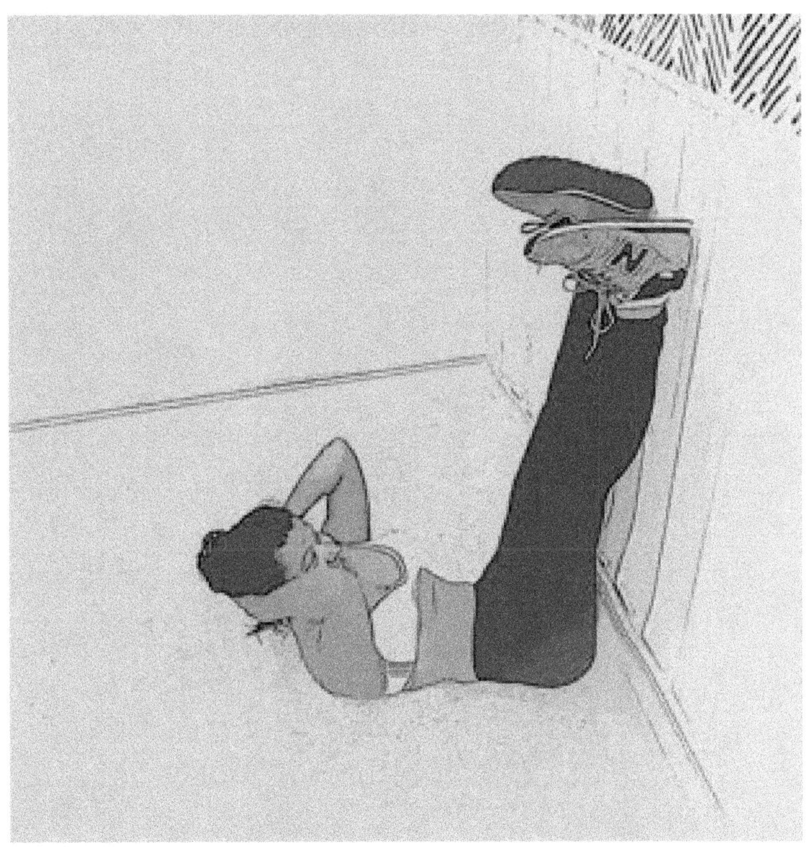

Abdominal Curl - Part 2: Curl torso towards knees, engaging abs.

* * *

4th minute: Advanced - Balance/Stability - Wall Handstand

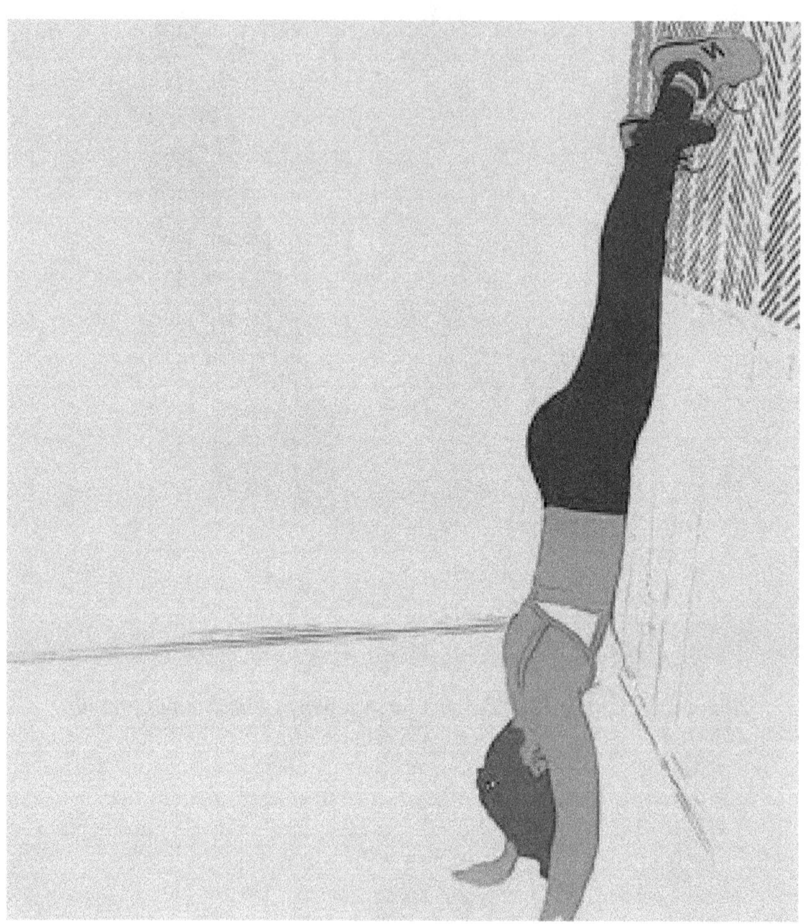

Wall Handstand: Kick up into a handstand against the wall, aim to balance without touching the wall, hold position.

* * *

5th minute: Advanced - Balance/Stability - Wall One-Arm Handstand

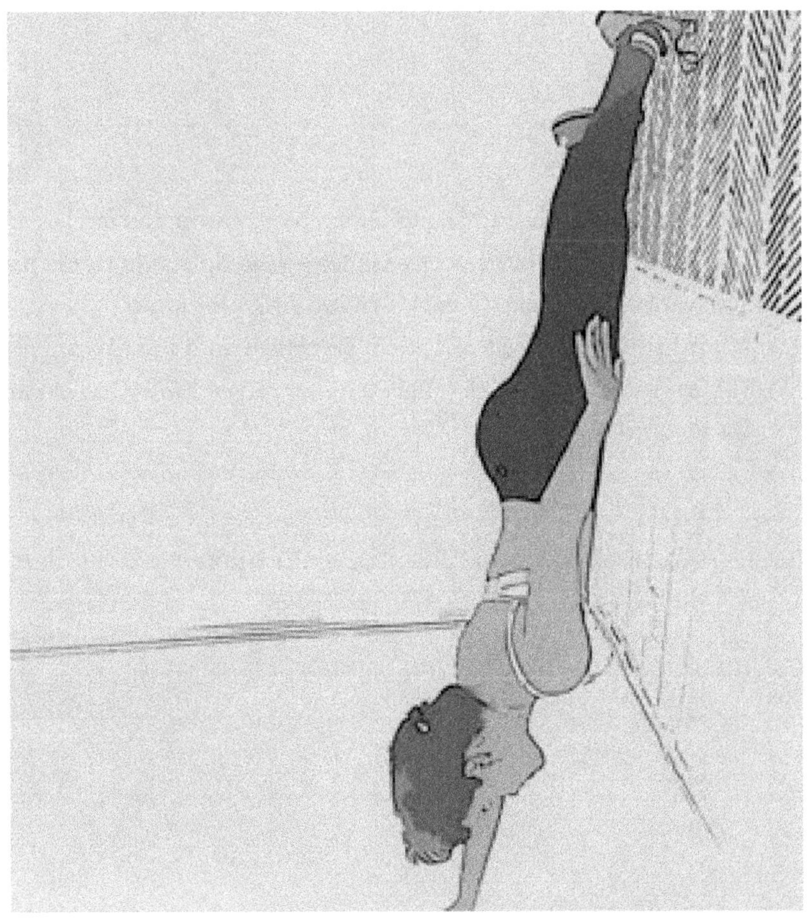

Wall One-Arm Handstand: In a wall handstand, shift weight to one arm, carefully lift the other arm off the wall, hold balance.

Advanced Tuesday

- **1st minute**: Advanced - Legs/Glutes - **Wall Jump Squats**
- **2nd minute**: Advanced - Legs/Glutes - **Wall Split Squat Jump**
- **3rd minute**: Advanced - Back - **Inverted Wall Plank**
- **4th minute**: Advanced - Back - **Wall Handstand Push-Up**
- **5th minute**: Advanced - Balance/Stability - **Wall One-Arm Handstand**

See Illustrations and How to Perform Exercise below

***

1st minute: Advanced - Legs/Glutes - Wall Jump Squats

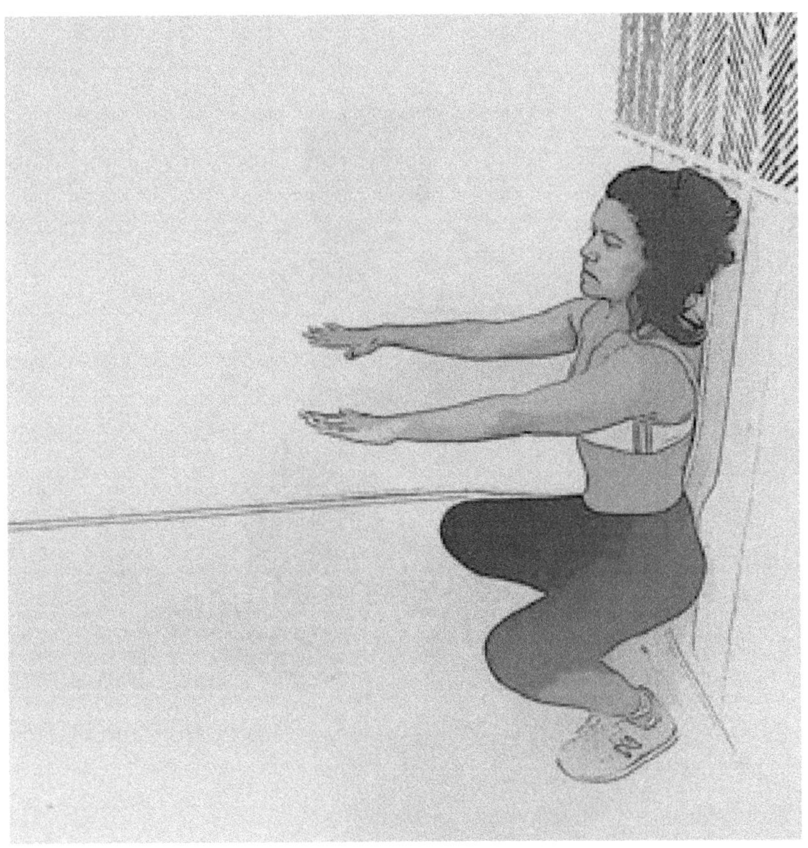

Wall Jump Squats: With back against the wall, lower into a squat, then jump up powerfully, land back in squat position.

* * *

2nd minute: Advanced - Legs/Glutes - Wall Split Squat Jump

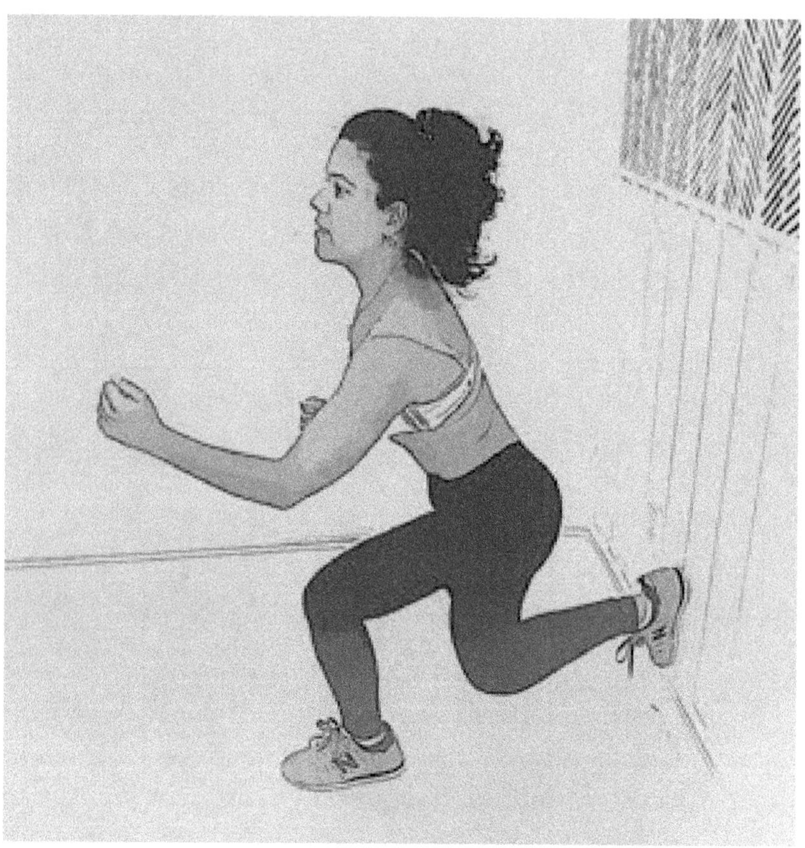

Wall Sit Squat Jump: Start with one leg on the wall behind you, jump and switch legs in a split squat motion, land softly.

* * *

3rd minute: Advanced - Back - Inverted Wall Plank

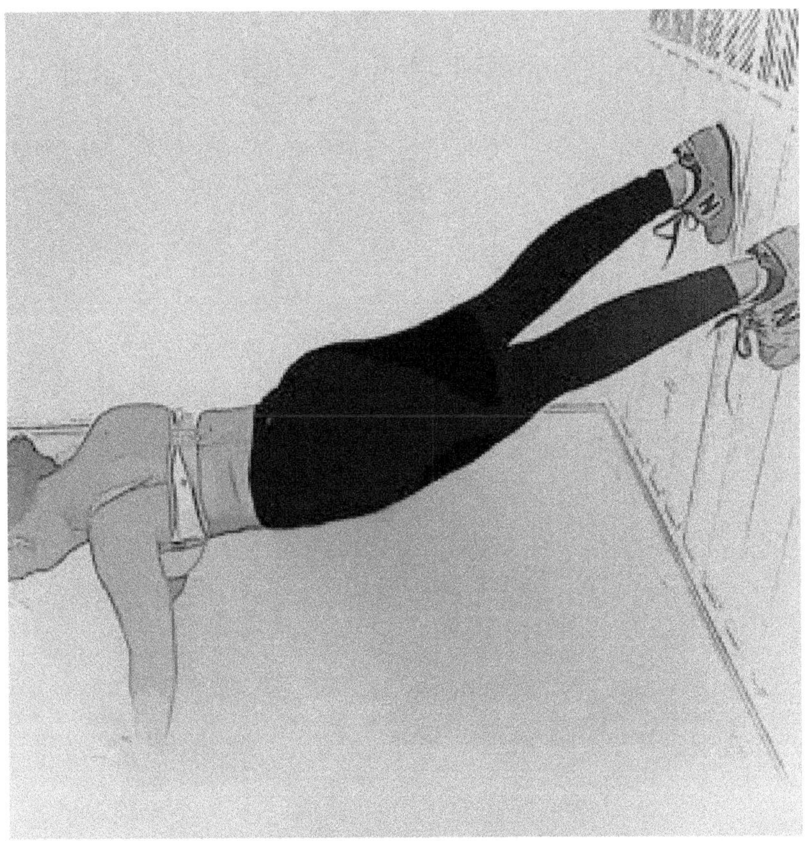

Inverted Wall Plank: With feet next to base of wall, kick into a plank position with hands straight to floor, feet braced on wall. Head should be in line with back and legs as straight as a board. For advancement, as shown above, elevate feet higher up wall while keeping that straight board formation.

* * *

4th minute: Advanced - Back - Wall Handstand Push-Up

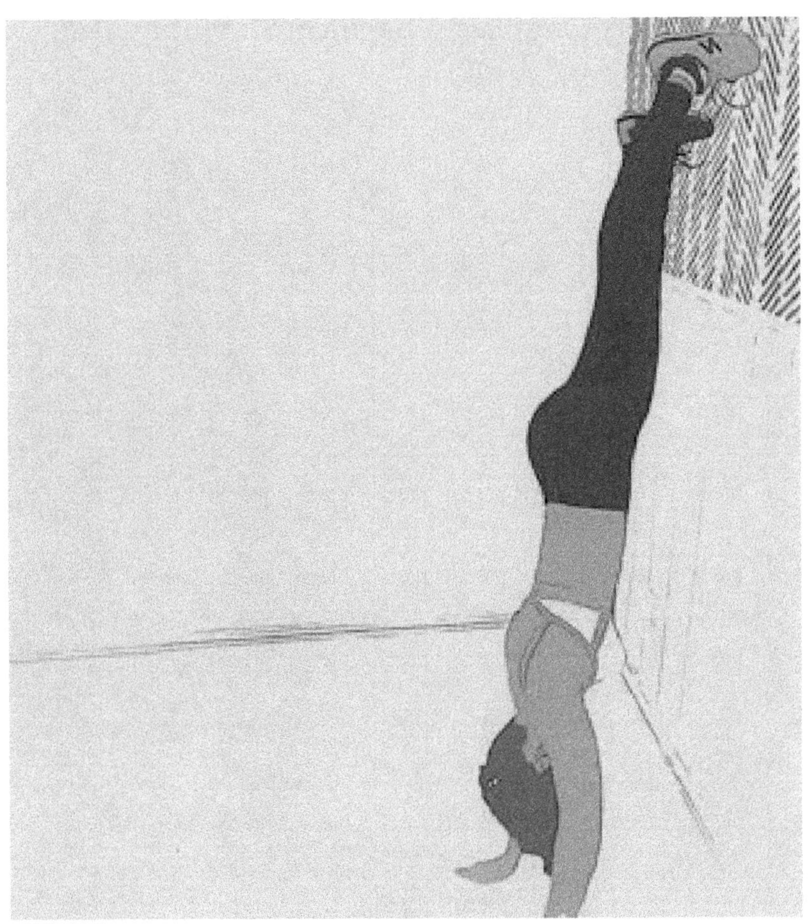

Wall Handstand Push-up: In a handstand against the wall, lower head towards ground by bending elbows, push back up.

* * *

5th minute: Advanced - Balance/Stability - Wall One-Arm Handstand

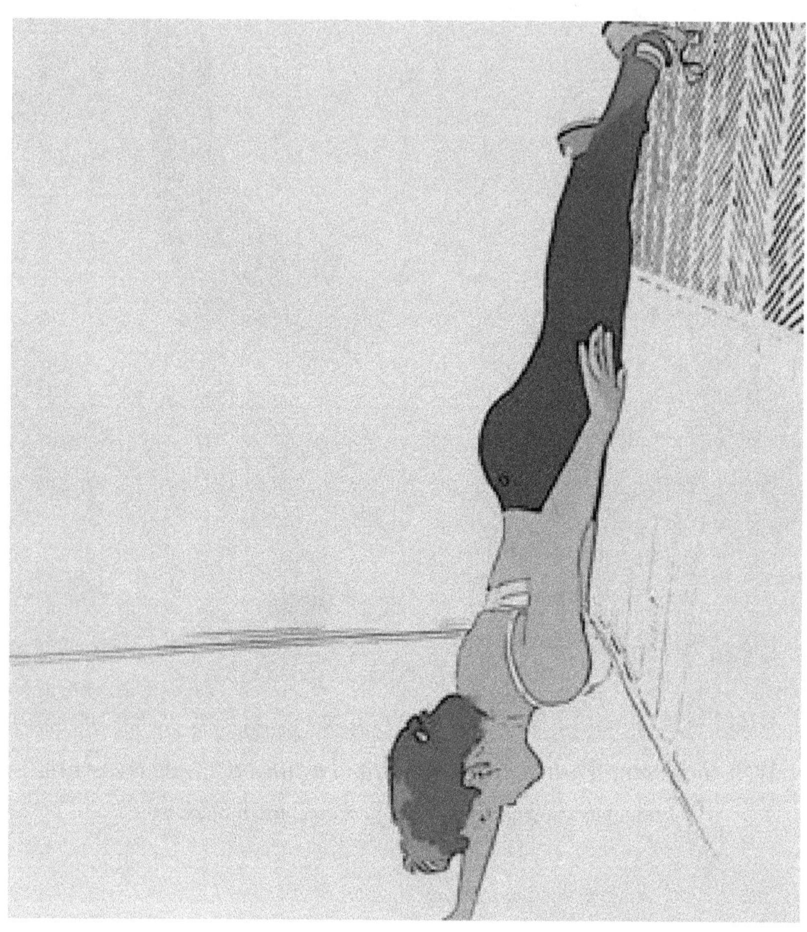

Wall One-Arm Handstand: In a wall handstand, shift weight to one arm, carefully lift the other arm off the wall, hold balance.

123

Advanced Wednesday

- **1st minute**: Advanced - Upper Body - **Wall Handstand Push-Up**
- **2nd minute**: Advanced - Upper Body - **Inverted Wall Plank**
- **3rd minute**: Advanced - Flexibility/Mobility - **Wall Oversplits**
- **4th minute**: Advanced - Flexibility/Mobility - **Wall Backbend**
- **5th minute**: Advanced - Full Body Integration - **Wall Handstand with Leg Twists**

See Illustrations and How to Perform Exercise below

* * *

1st minute: Advanced - Upper Body - Wall Handstand Push-Up

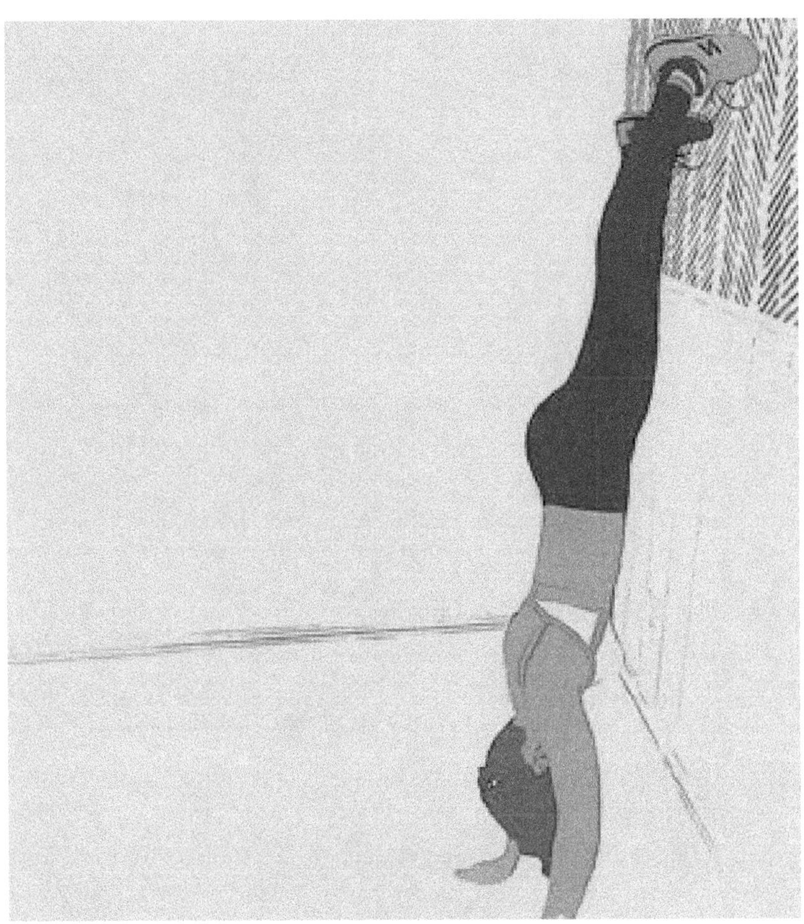

Wall Handstand Push-up: In a handstand against the wall, lower head towards ground by bending elbows, push back up.

* * *

2nd minute: Advanced - Upper Body - Inverted Wall Plank

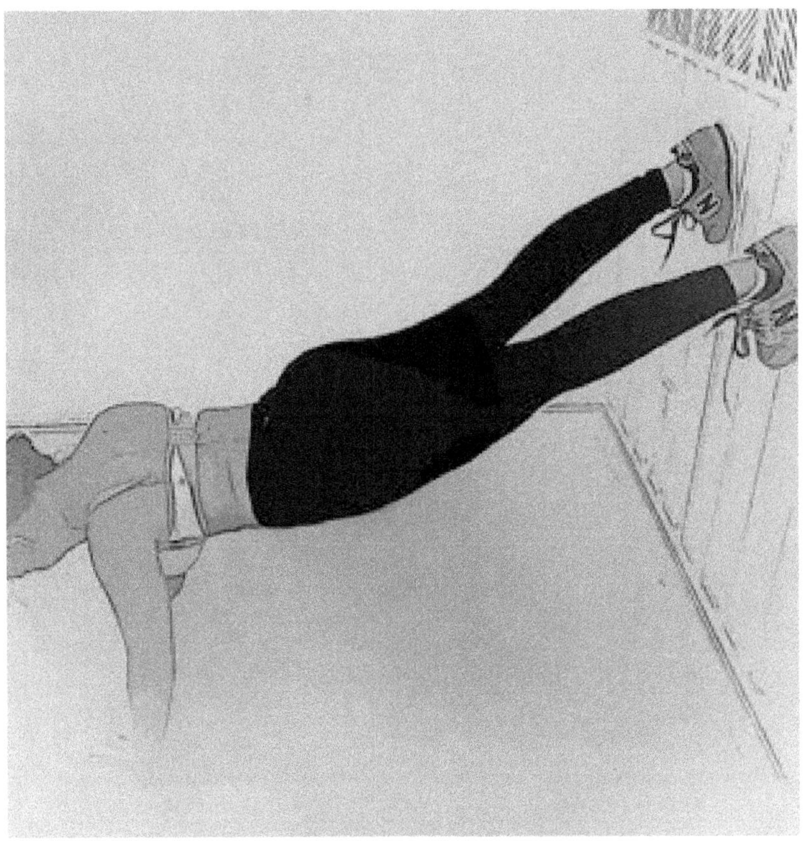

Inverted Wall Plank: With feet next to base of wall, kick into a plank position with hands straight to floor, feet braced on wall. Head should be in line with back and legs as straight as a board. For advancement, as shown above, elevate feet higher up wall while keeping that straight board formation.

* * *

3rd minute: Advanced - Flexibility/Mobility - Wall Oversplits

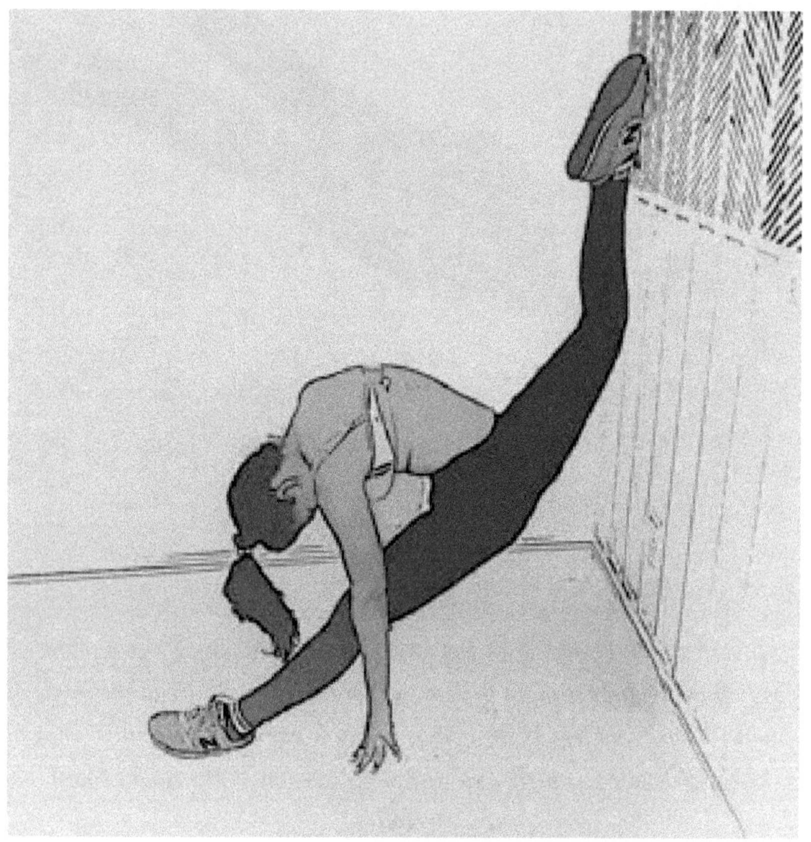

Wall Oversplits: Place one leg on the wall into an oversplit, keep the other leg on the ground, hold stretch.

* * *

4th minute: Advanced - Flexibility/Mobility - Wall Backbend

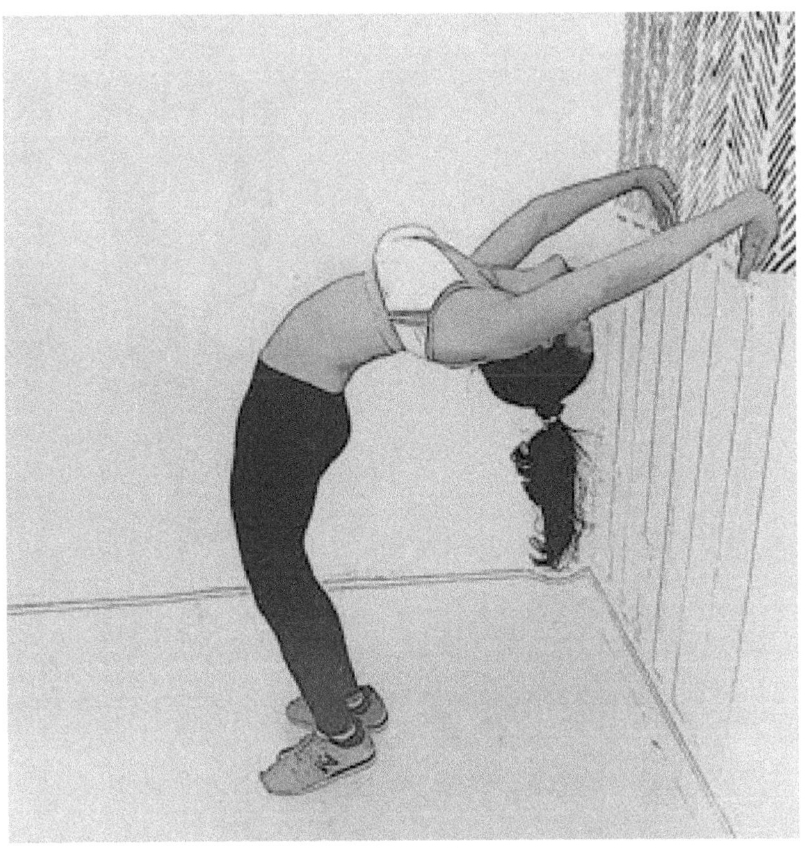

Wall Backbend: Stand facing away from the wall, reach hands back to touch the wall, push hips forward, arch into a backbend.

* * *

5th minute: Advanced - Full Body Integration - Wall Handstand with Leg Twists

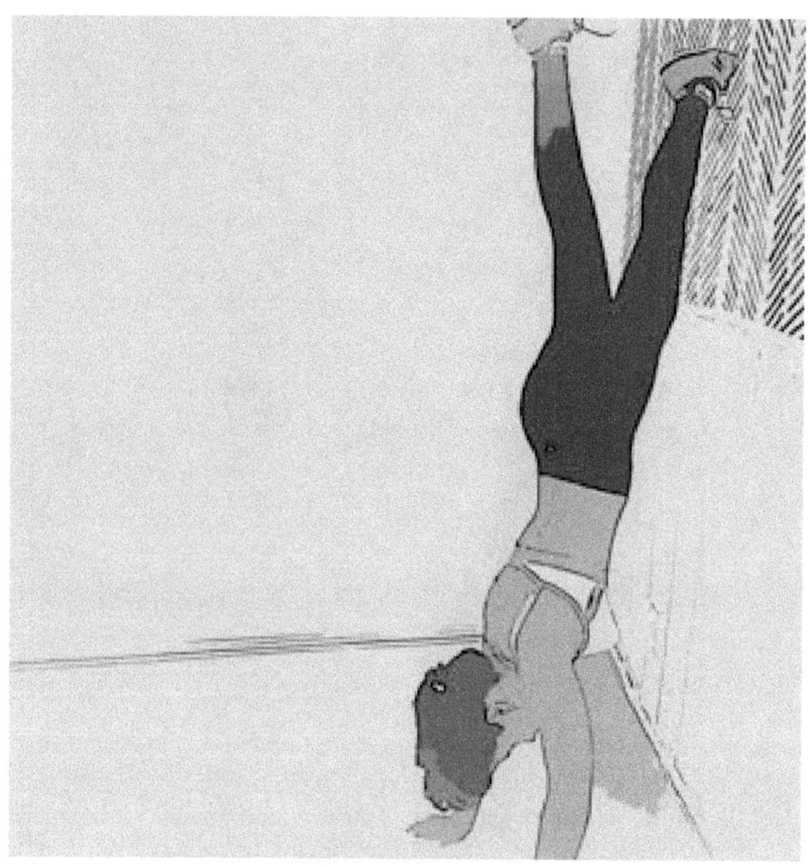

Wall Handstand with Leg Twists: In a handstand against the wall, twist legs side to side, maintaining control and balance.

Advanced Thursday

- **1st minute**: Advanced - Core/Abs - **Inverted Wall Mountain Climbers**
- **2nd minute**: Advanced - Core/Abs - **Wall Scissor Kicks**
- **3rd minute**: Advanced - Core/Abs - **Wall Abdominal Curl**
- **4th minute**: Advanced - Balance/Stability - **Wall Handstand**
- **5th minute**: Advanced - Balance/Stability - **Wall One-Arm Handstand**

See Illustrations and How to Perform Exercise below

* * *

1st minute: Advanced - Core/Abs - Inverted Wall Mountain Climbers

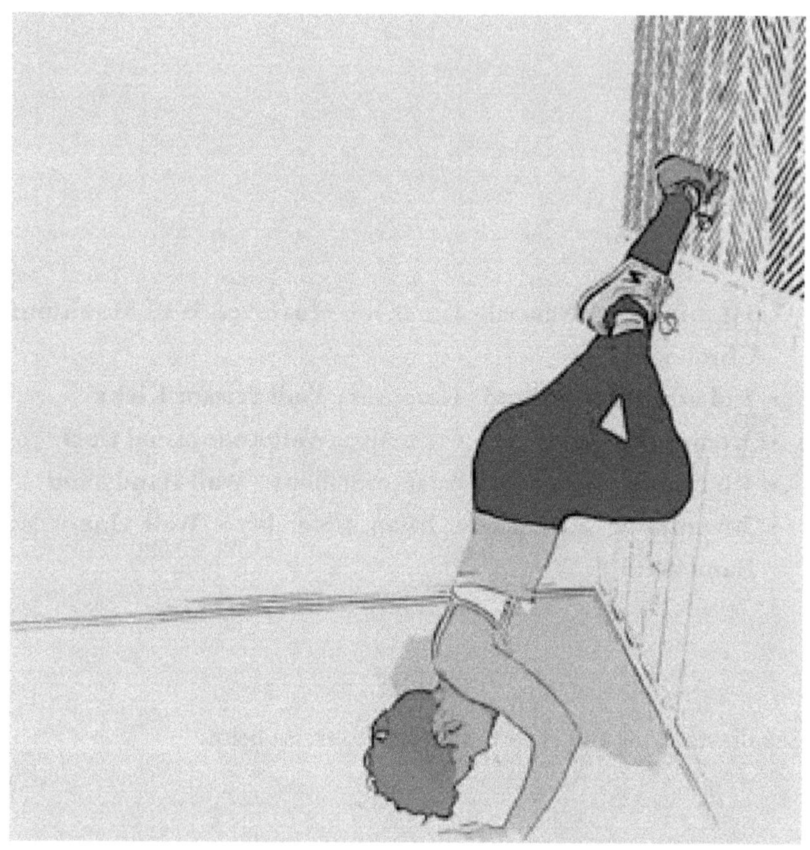

Inverted Wall Mountain Climbers: In a handstand against the wall, alternate driving knees towards chest in a controlled manner.

* * *

2nd minute: Advanced - Core/Abs - Wall Scissor Kicks

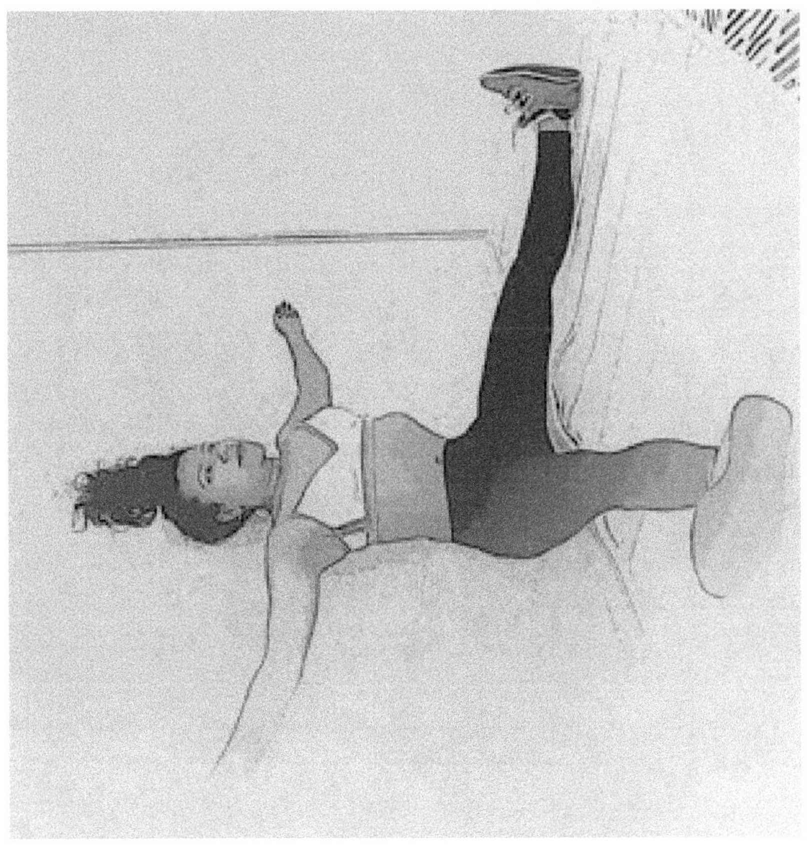

Wall Scissor Kicks: Lie on back, legs up against the wall, perform scissor kicks by alternating leg positions.

* * *

3rd minute: Advanced - Core/Abs - Wall Abdominal Curl

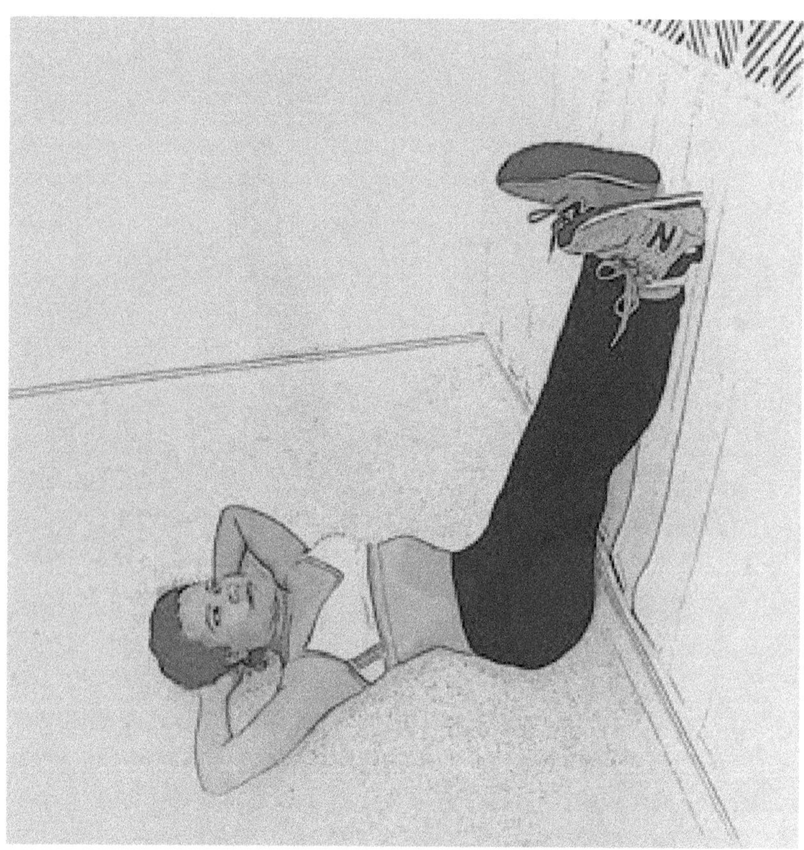

Abdominal Curl - Part 1: Lay down with back against the floor, buttocks on the wall with legs extending vertically along wall toward ceiling.

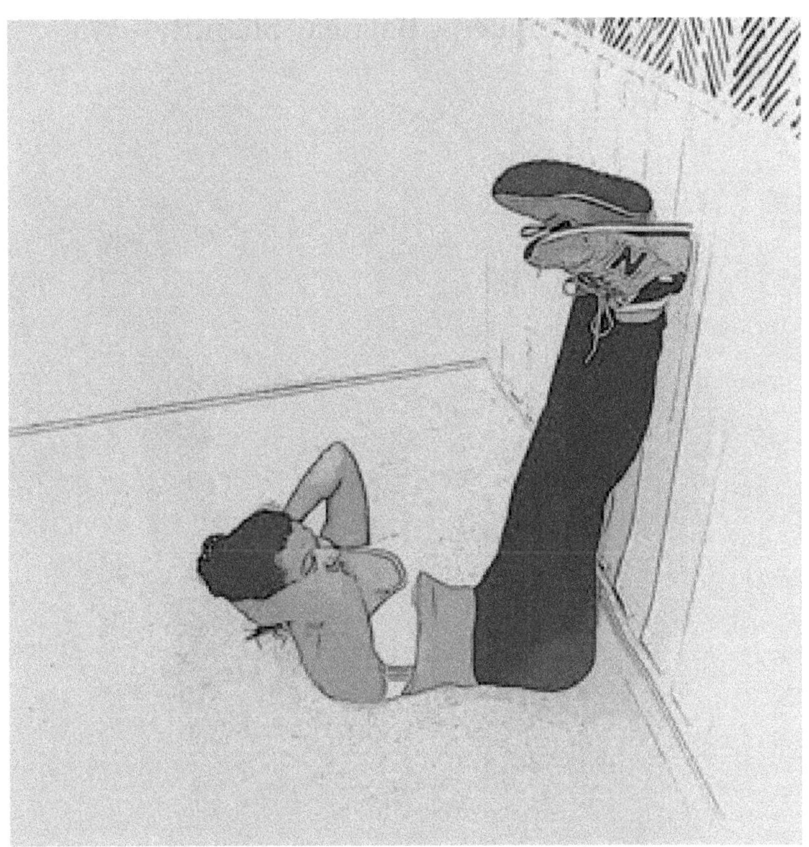

Abdominal Curl - Part 2: Curl torso towards knees, engaging abs.

* * *

4th minute: Advanced - Balance/Stability - Wall Handstand

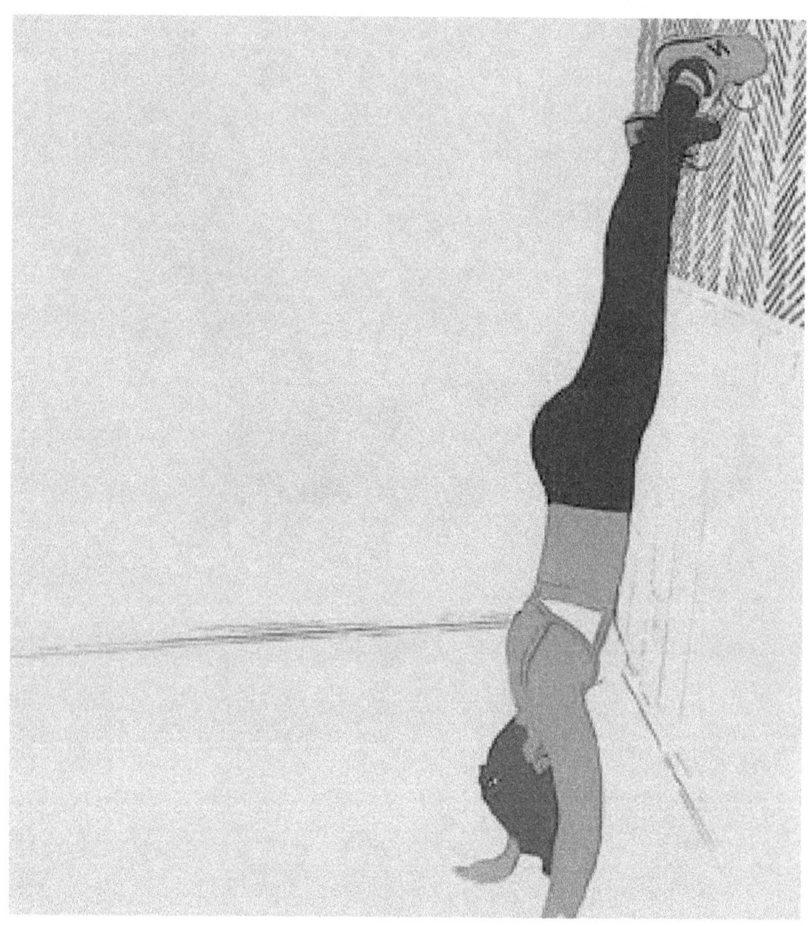

Wall Handstand: Kick up into a handstand against the wall, aim to balance without touching the wall, hold position.

* * *

5th minute: Advanced - Balance/Stability - Wall One-Arm Handstand

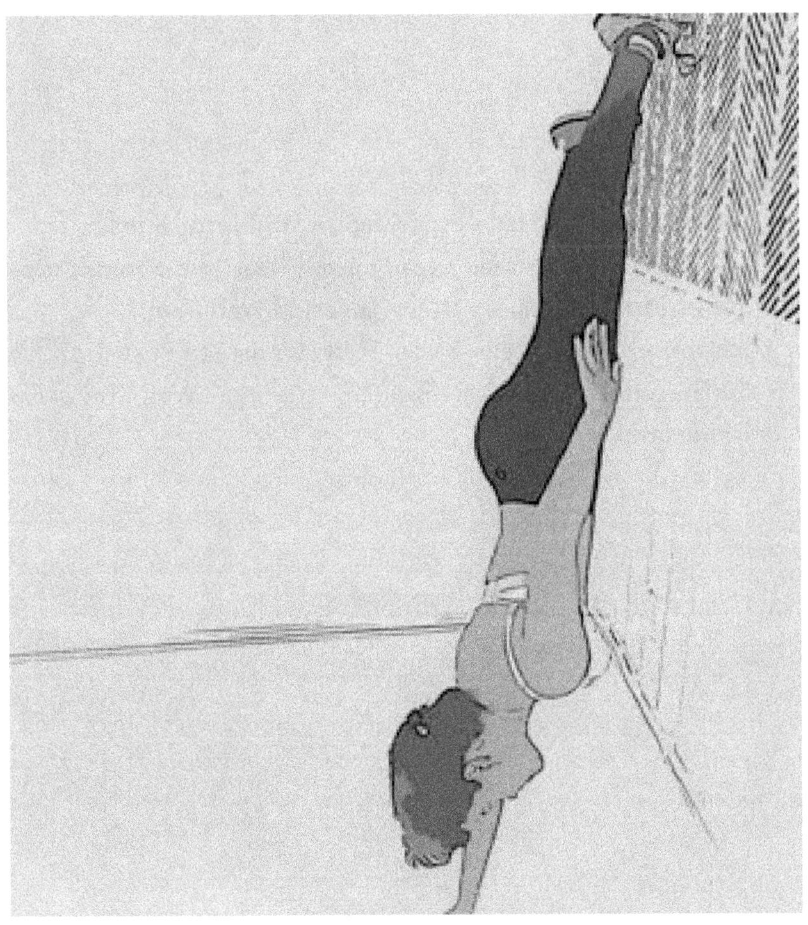

Wall One-Arm Handstand: In a wall handstand, shift weight to one arm, carefully lift the other arm off the wall, hold balance.

Advanced Friday

- **1st minute**: Advanced - Legs/Glutes - **Wall Jump Squats**
- **2nd minute**: Advanced - Legs/Glutes - **Wall Split Squat Jump**
- **3rd minute**: Advanced - Back - **Inverted Wall Plank**
- **4th minute**: Advanced - Back - **Wall Handstand Push-Up**
- **5th minute**: Advanced - Balance/Stability - **Wall One-Arm Handstand**

See Illustrations and How to Perform Exercise below

* * *

1st minute: Advanced - Legs/Glutes - Wall Jump Squats

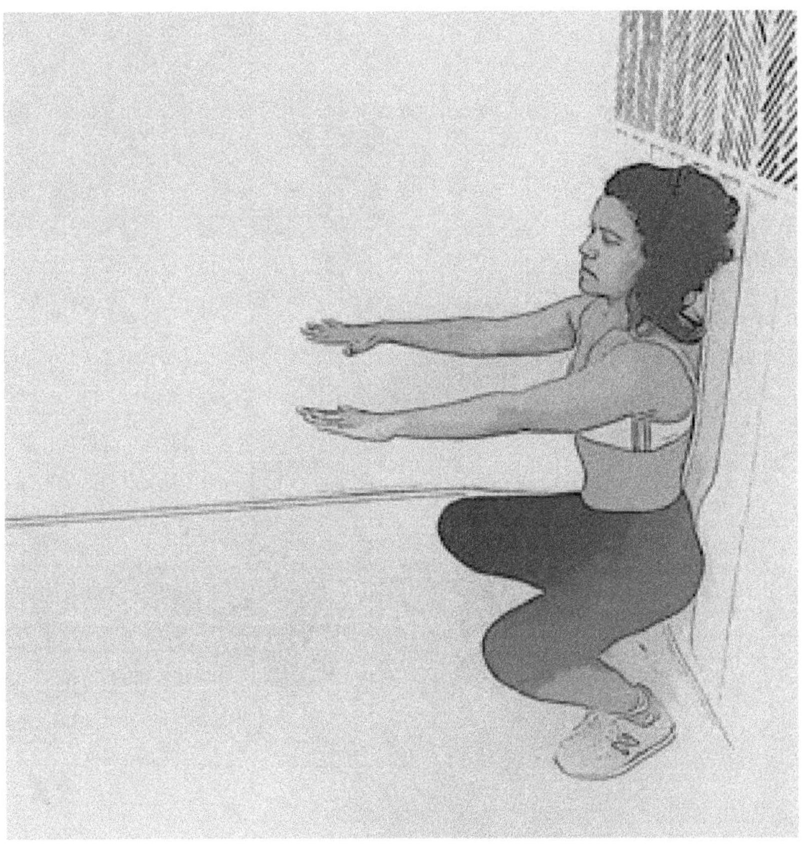

Wall Jump Squats: With back against the wall, lower into a squat, then jump up powerfully, land back in squat position.

* * *

2nd minute: Advanced - Legs/Glutes - Wall Split Squat Jump

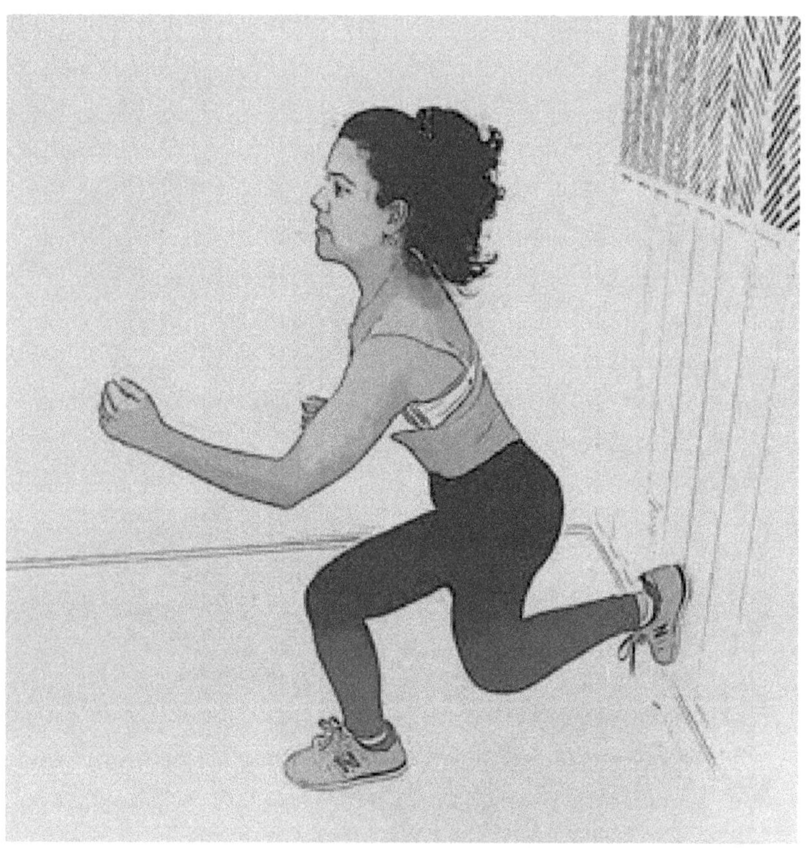

Wall Sit Squat Jump: Start with one leg on the wall behind you, jump and switch legs in a split squat motion, land softly.

* * *

3rd minute: Advanced - Back - Inverted Wall Plank

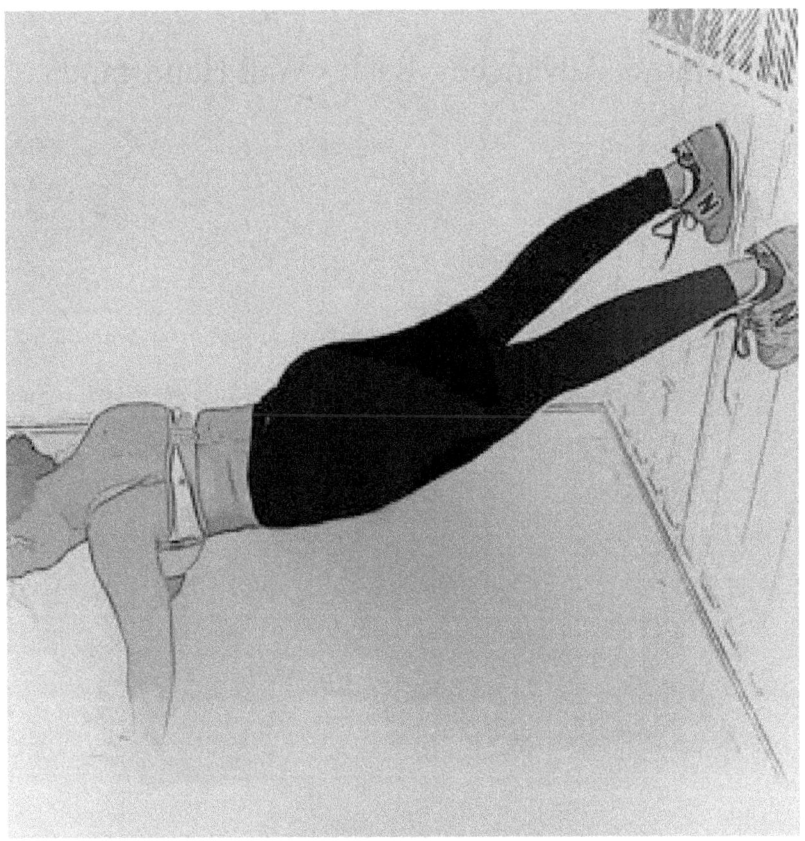

Inverted Wall Plank: With feet next to base of wall, kick into a plank position with hands straight to floor, feet braced on wall. Head should be in line with back and legs as straight as a board. For advancement, as shown above, elevate feet higher up wall while keeping that straight board formation.

* * *

4th minute: Advanced - Back - Wall Handstand Push-Up

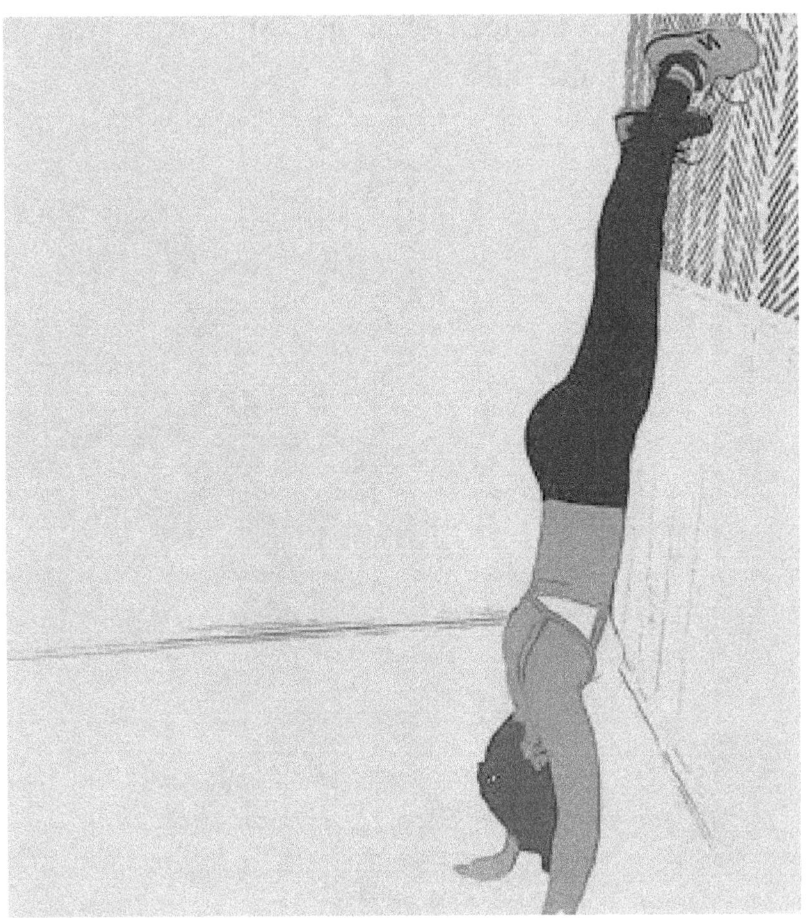

Wall Handstand Push-up: In a handstand against the wall, lower head towards ground by bending elbows, push back up.

* * *

5th minute: Advanced - Balance/Stability - Wall One-Arm Handstand

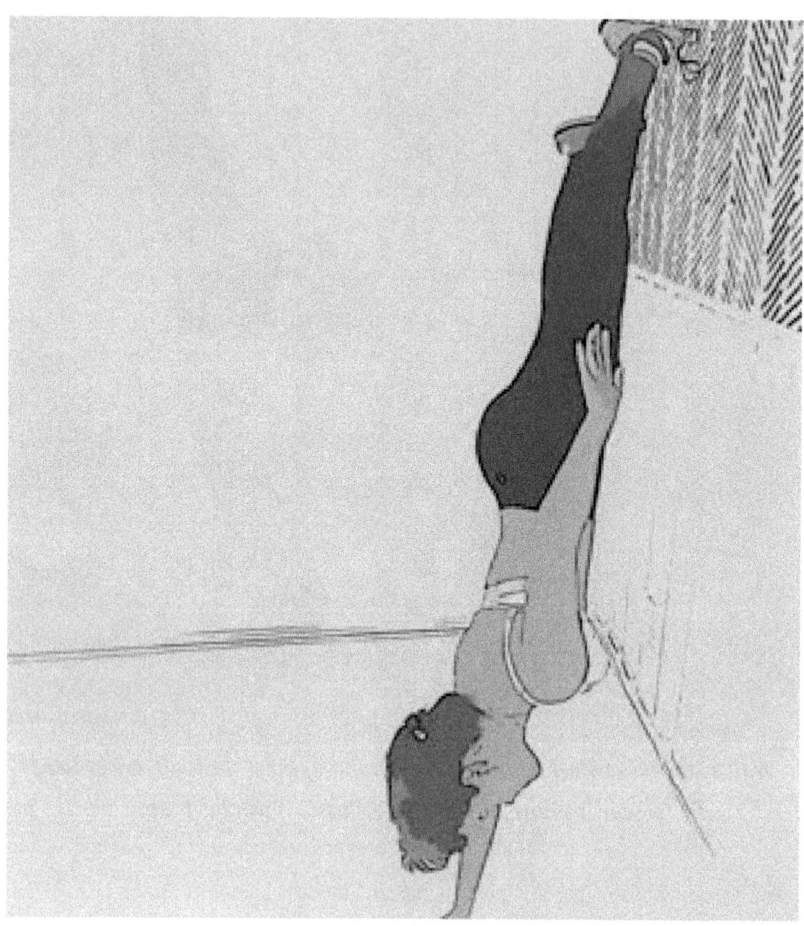

Wall One-Arm Handstand: In a wall handstand, shift weight to one arm, carefully lift the other arm off the wall, hold balance.

145

Advanced Saturday

- **1st minute**: Advanced - Upper Body - **Wall Handstand Push-Up**
- **2nd minute**: Advanced - Upper Body - **Inverted Wall Plank**
- **3rd minute**: Advanced - Flexibility/Mobility - **Wall Oversplits**
- **4th minute**: Advanced - Flexibility/Mobility - **Wall Backbend**
- **5th minute**: Advanced - Full Body Integration - **Wall Handstand with Leg Twists**

See Illustrations and How to Perform Exercise below

*　*　*

1st minute: Advanced - Upper Body - Wall Handstand Push-Up

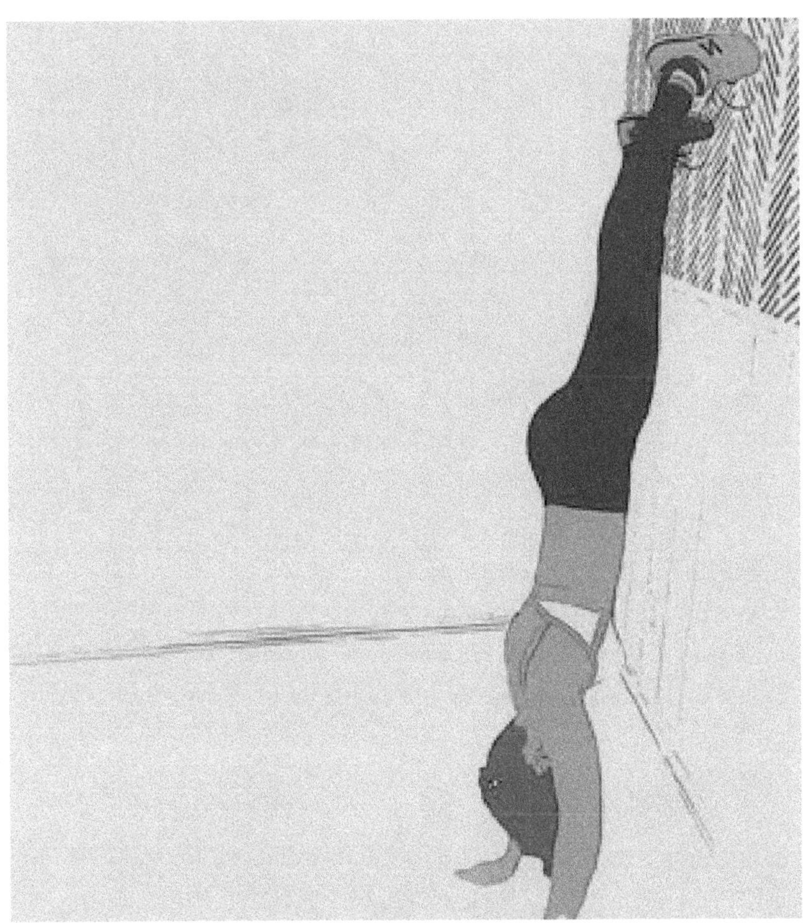

Wall Handstand Push-up: In a handsatnd against the wall, lower head towards ground by bending elbows, push back up.

* * *

2nd minute: Advanced - Upper Body - Inverted Wall Plank

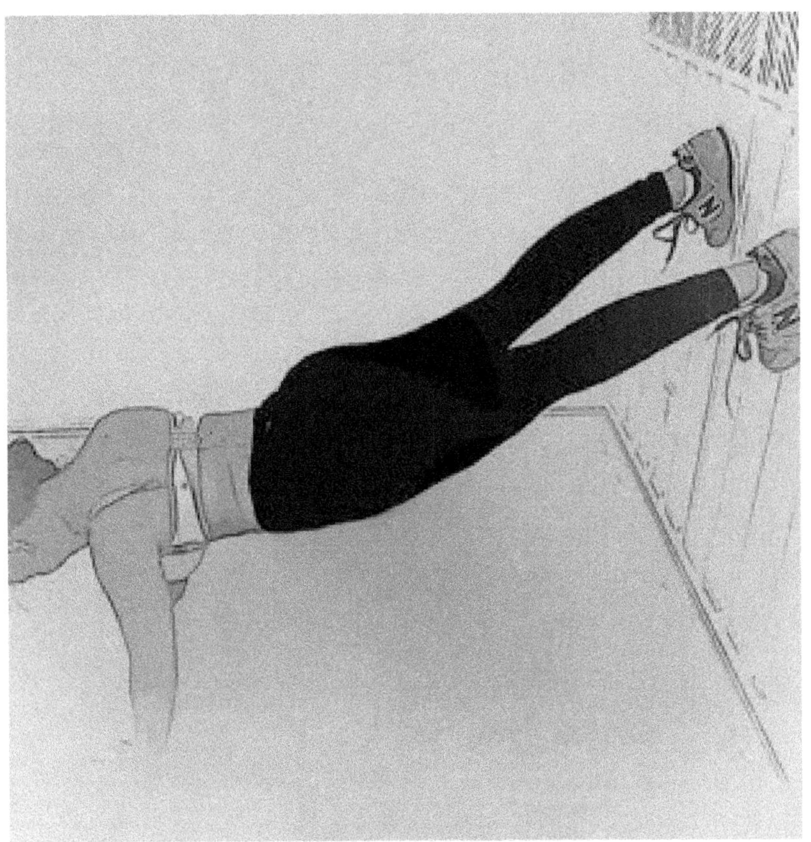

Inverted Wall Plank: With feet next to base of wall, kick into a plank position with hands straight to floor, feet braced on wall. Head should be in line with back and legs as straight as a board. For advancement, as shown above, elevate feet higher up wall while keeping that straight board formation.

* * *

3rd minute: Advanced - Flexibility/Mobility - Wall Oversplits

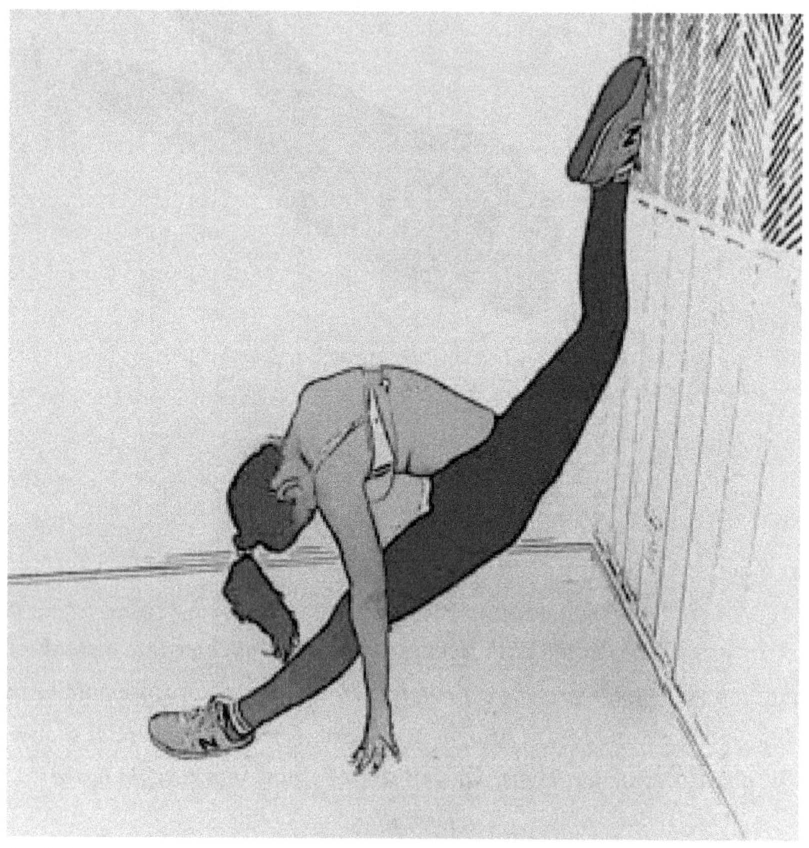

Wall Oversplits: Place one leg on the wall into an oversplit, keep the other leg on the ground, hold stretch.

* * *

4th minute: Advanced - Flexibility/Mobility - Wall Backbend

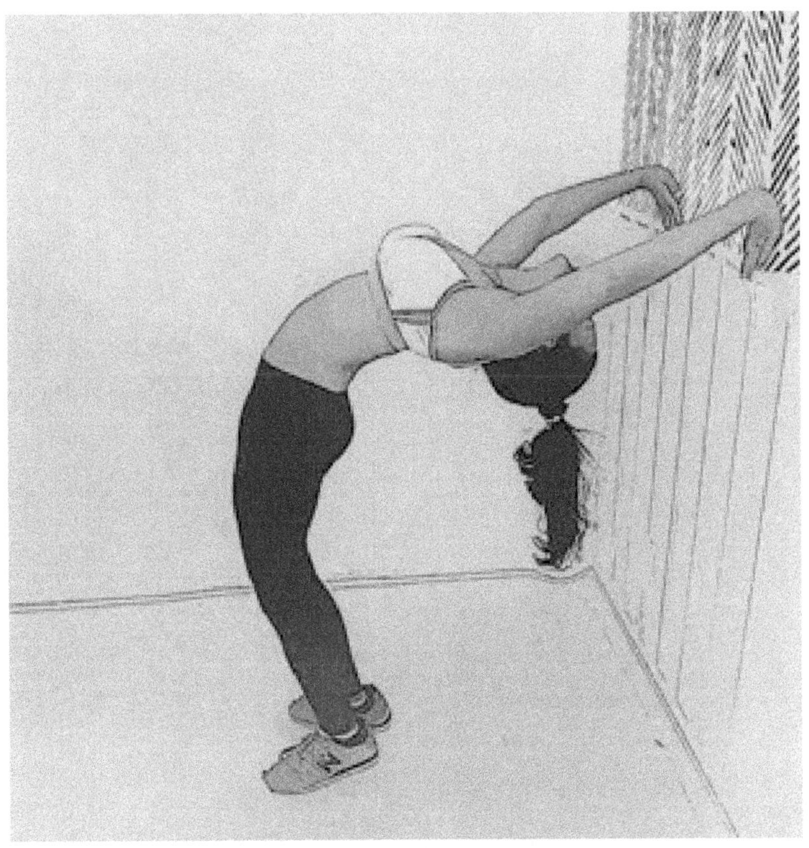

Wall Backbend: Stand facing away from the wall, reach hands back to touch the wall, push hips forward, arch into a backbend.

* * *

5th minute: Advanced - Full Body Integration - Wall Handstand with Leg Twists

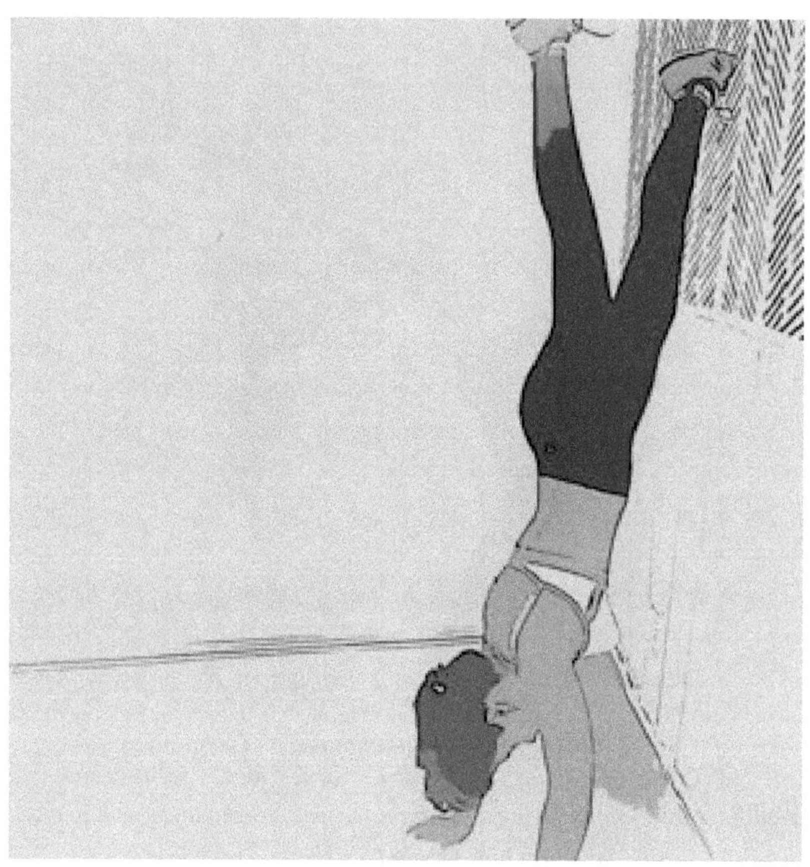

Wall Handstand with Leg Twists: In a handstand against the wall, twist legs side to side, maintaining control and balance.

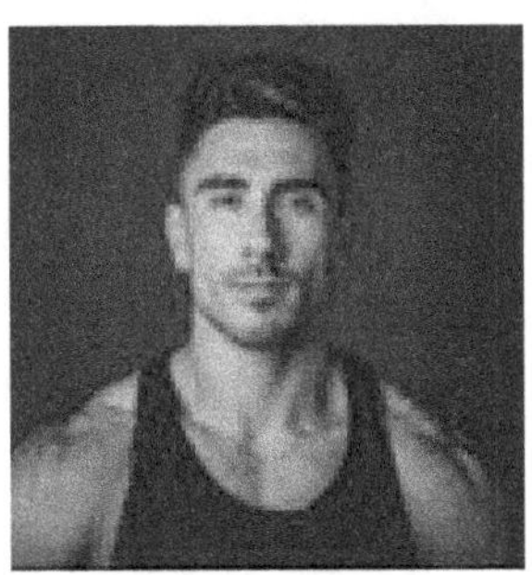

About the Author

Bronco Porter is an inspiring 34-year-old father of two who is highly passionate about his work as a fitness instructor, wellness coach, and author.

He is committed to providing exercises that are easy to follow and can be done with minimal equipment. With his extensive knowledge and experience, Bronco is now writing multiple books focusing on Pilates and Calisthenics, offering guidance on techniques, benefits, and routines tailored for busy individuals.

Bronco's mission is to make exercises more accessible and appealing to everyone, regardless of their fitness level. His goal is to help as many people as possible to achieve a stronger core, improved posture, and a balanced mind-body connection.

His enthusiasm and passion for Wall Pilates are contagious, and his books will sure to be the go-to resource for those looking to integrate this effective workout into their busy schedules.